I0868223

The Covert Life of Hospital Architecture

The Covert Life of Hospital Architecture

Julie Zook and Kerstin Sailer

UCLPRESS

First published in 2022 by
UCL Press
University College London
Gower Street
London WC1E 6BT

Available to download free: www.uclpress.co.uk

A CIP catalogue record for this book is available from The British Library.

ISBN: 978-1-80008-090-4 (Hbk.)
ISBN: 978-1-80008-089-8 (Pbk.)
ISBN: 978-1-80008-088-1 (PDF)
ISBN: 978-1-80008-091-1 (epub)
ISBN: 978-1-80008-092-8 (mobi)
DOI: https://doi.org/10.14324/111.9781800080881

Julie:
For Ezra, Sofia and Nathan

Kerstin:
For Danah, Victoria and Christian

Contents

List of figures xiii
List of contributors xix
Acknowledgements ix
Foreword - Jerri Brittin xxi

Chapter 1: The spatial dimension of hospital life
Julie Zook 1

Chapter 2: Pillow
Introduction – *Julie Zook* 21
The patient and the reciprocal view – *Michelle Ossmann* 22
Response Essay: The evolution of surveillance in ICU design – *George Tingwald* 41

Chapter 3: Table
Introduction – *Julie Zook* 55
Working together in healthcare space – *Rosica Pachilova and Kerstin Sailer* 56
Response Essay: Spatial intelligence to support a team-of-teams ecosystem – relevance and need in practice – *Upali Nanda* 80

Chapter 4: Hallway
Introduction – *Julie Zook* 92
The visitor and hospital corridor design – *Julie Zook and Sonit Bafna* 93
Response Essay: Designing a human-centred hospital wayfinding system – *Carlo Giannasca* 117

Chapter 5: Outlook
The social logic of spaces for health: The relational hospital as a response to COVID-19 – *Kerstin Sailer* 130

Index 158

Acknowledgements

Teaching is said to detract from writing, but the students in my college have inspired me, helped me and made the work pleasant. My graduate students, present and past, brought curiosity, energy and clarity to design and analysis of healthcare spaces that kept me going me when I was running on fumes. Spencer Reddick, Maria Leon, Karla Perez, Rebecca Barnes, Lauren Hunter, Daniel Rios, Victor Carrillo, Kam Ambler and Meagan Matthews assisted with research and graphic production in important ways.

This book was conceptualized just prior to COVID-19 and will be published as the pandemic goes on its third year. The world changed around this project, and architects are now more aware that individual health is conditioned by physical and social contexts that are more extensive and complex than any given building. Health problems are social problems, but the implications of the social dimension of health for architecture are not yet clear. This book picks up a corner of the problem by focusing on techniques for the social and functional life of hospitals. It builds on sociological theories and building morphological approaches including those of Émile Durkheim, Mary Douglas, Bill Hillier, and Michael Benedikt.

The Texas Tech University and College of Architecture provided generous financial support for early research that led to this book. Additionally, the Texas Tech Humanities Center channelled a constant flow of new perspectives that helped me sharpen my own. I am particularly appreciative for the Humanities Center Alumni College Fellowship that supported my writing.

My work with BSA LifeStructures has been essential to being able to think critically and in detail about how research meets practice. Getting to better know the specific problems that clients and architects face has been invaluable. I especially thank Tim Spence, Teri Joy, Jennifer Worley, Monte Hoover, Chase Miller and Melanie Harris for their collegiality as I look forward to our ongoing collaboration.

Chris Penfold at UCL Press and anonymous peer reviewers supported our main aims, while presenting invaluable questions, suggestions and criticisms.

From where I sit, this edited volume resembles a small get-together with a mix of old friends and new acquaintances. For some of us, the book is the extended form of a conversation about what is going on with research and healthcare architecture that we have been having for years through telephone calls, shared projects and conversations at conference venues. This is a book of research, but in making it, we wanted to speak with practising architects and designers, the clients and publics with whom they seek solutions, and the students who will in time enter these areas of practice. What I am saying is that making esoteric ideas more accessible is at the centre of this project, and it is for this reason that we are particularly pleased and proud to publish this book open access.

Julie Zook

An African proverb suggests that it takes a village to raise a child. Something similar could probably be said about research in general, and the process of editing and writing a book. Many people have joined me on my journey from architecture school, throughout my PhD, then oscillating between workplace consultancy and academic scholarship to my position now at the Bartlett School of Architecture at UCL.

While still in architecture school, Barbara Zibell fuelled my curiosity for the social side of architecture and the impact that spatial design has on human behaviours. During my early research on workplaces and office buildings, I came across Space Syntax and, like many others, I was intrigued by its possibilities and methodological rigour. Bill Hillier accepted my application to join the Space Syntax Lab as a visiting PhD student with a graceful one-liner email, sent within an hour of my request. It is fair to say that I owe my love of data to Alan Penn with whom I spent many long hours discussing research ideas and looking through spreadsheets.

In expanding my understanding of places of work, from offices to other building types, Ray Pradinuk was instrumental – a graduate from one of the first cohorts of the Space Syntax master's programme at UCL, long before my time there. More than 10 years ago, in 2011, we met in London to plot and plan a research project on outpatient clinics, which eventually took us to the Netherlands to study best practice examples. From then on, I was hooked on the topic of hospital architecture and design.

Working with colleagues as well as my PhD students at the Bartlett School of Architecture has broadened my horizon significantly.

Collaborating with Rosica Pachilova on communication in hospital wards has been fun and fruitful, winning us the RIBA President's Award for research in 2019. A project on the potential spread of pathogens in hospital wards funded by the Arts and Humanities Research Council in 2018–19 highlighted the power of co-design and raising awareness among healthcare workers. Accompanying my colleague Julia Backhaus into wards, dressed in a self-designed superbug costume to engage healthcare workers in conversations taught me that research comes in many different forms and shapes.

Finally, working with Julie Zook and our fantastic group of authors featured in this book has been a rewarding experience. Bridging between academia and practice and offering a fresh perspective on hospital architecture, revealing its intrinsic social logic and its usability is what inspired this book. We hope that it will inspire you as a reader as well.

Kerstin Sailer

List of figures

1.1	The transparent architecture of the Pioneer Health Centre, 1935 Dell & Wainwright/RIBA Collections.	7
1.2	Unpartitioned space at the Pioneer Health Centre, Dell & Wainwright/RIBA Collections.	8
1.3	Pioneer Health Centre sections, as drawn by Victor Carrillo and Daniel Rios, 2021.	9
1.4	Pioneer Health Centre floorplan, as drawn by Victor Carrillo and Daniel Rios, 2021. The first floor (one level above ground) has lounge and cafeteria spaces on the long arms of the plan, overlooks recreation spaces on the short arms, and has the pool at the centre.	9
1.5	Dr Reed's sketch plan of Surgicenter, Wood Library, Museum of Anesthesiology.	11
1.6	The Surgicenter floorplan and elevation, reprinted from the *Journal of Pediatric Surgery*, Vol 7, Daniel T. Cloud, Wallace A. Reed, John L. Ford, Laurence M. Linkner, David S. Trump and George W. Dorman, 'The surgicenter: A fresh concept in outpatient pediatric surgery' (1972), 207, with permission from Elsevier.	12
2.1	The patient-nurse visual link is critical for safety, but it has been difficult to fully understand how it works. Drawn by Victor Carrillo and Daniel Rios, 2021.	24
2.2a and 2.2b	From the patient head of bed, different conditions for patient visibility. Drawn by Victor Carrillo and Daniel Rios, 2021.	25

2.3	Isovist polygons (360°) as described by Benedikt (1979); generated from a patient bed (black point, grey field) and a nurse station (blue point and field). Drawn by Victor Carrillo and Daniel Rios, 2021.	30
2.4	Visual connectivity graph example. Drawn by Victor Carrillo and Daniel Rios, 2021.	31
2.5a and 2.5b	Concept diagram of the principle of isovist connectivity. The purple area is visible from the patient head of bed, while the blue is the area that can see some part of the purple. The larger the overall area, the better the capacity of the nurse to keep the patient in view while remaining visually connected to the rest of the unit. Diagram by Victor Carrillo and Daniel Rios, 2021.	35
2.6	Visual connectivity graphs for four Emory intensive care units (ICUs): Unit A (top left) B (top right) and C and D (bottom row). Image by Michelle Ossmann, 2015.	37
2.7	High (green), medium (gold) and low (red) isovist connectivity values for patient rooms in four ICUs. Image by Victor Carrillo and Daniel Rios, 2021.	38
2.8	Nurse sub-station and visibility to patient rooms. Courtesy of Stanford Health Care.	43
2.9	Charting alcoves and visibility to patient rooms. Courtesy of Stanford Health Care.	44
2.10	The charting alcoves were particularly useful during pandemic conditions. Courtesy of Stanford Health Care, image by Will Pryce.	46
2.11	Patient rooms with outside views and places for extended community. Courtesy of Stanford Health Care, image by Will Pryce.	46
3.1	Working side-by-side or teamwork in a nurse station? Drawn by Victor Carrillo and Daniel Rios, 2021.	57
3.2	*Florence Nightingale*, image credit: Jess Sweeney through Wikimedia Commons.	59
3.3	Florence Nightingale's diagram of the causes of mortality in the army, 1820–1910. Image credit: Wikimedia Commons.	62

3.4	A Nightingale ward at St Thomas's Hospital, 1900. Image credit: Augustine Rischgitz via Wikimedia Commons.	63
3.5a and 3.5b	Studies in space required for nurses to make a bed (left) and set up an intravenous transfusion (right).	64
3.6	Mapping student nurse travel, 1955. By kind permission of the Trustees of University College London Hospitals NHS Foundation Trust.	65
3.7	Concept diagram showing the principle of accumulated visual exposure for a typical nurse task path. For the SCI, the sum of exposure for task paths are multiplied by estimated task frequency. Concept diagram by Victor Carrillo and Daniel Rios, 2021.	72
3.8	Visual connectivity graphs for 100 per cent single-room wards, with SCI values listed. Image by Rosica Pachilova, 2019.	74
3.9	The SCI of UK inpatient wards, with National Health Service Care Quality Ratings, and wards with 100 per cent single-patient rooms called out. Image by Rosica Pachilova, 2019.	75
3.10	Layout strategies tested for effect on SCI. (1) Increased corridor width by 50 cm; (2) Enlarged open space at corridor crossings with high visual connectivity; and (3) Change nurse assignment from centralised (left) to decentralised (right) nurse-station model and vice versa. Image by Rosica Pachilova, 2019, redrawn by Victor Carrillo and Daniel Rios, 2021.	77
3.11	Promedica inpatient tower design after using spatial analytics to reduce hide-away spaces, increase peer-peer and patient-provider visibility, and reduce wasted walking, 2020. Copyright HKS Architects.	82
3.12	A layered mapping tool to link spatial and human analytics from Soleimani, Nanda and Augustine, 2020. Copyright HKS Architects.	83
4.1	A well-designed hospital with a challenging corridor system. Tsoi Kobus, used with permission, 2021.	103

4.2	Diagrammatic redrawing of hospital corridor plan.	104
4.3	The plan and corridor system at Rikshospitalet. Drawn by Victor Carrillo and Daniel Rios, 2021.	107
4.4	Diagrammatic redrawing of Rikshospitalet corridor plan.	107
4.5	A hospital corridor that downplays its institutional function. Drawn by Victor Carrillo and Daniel Rios, 2021.	108
4.6	A floorplan of the Gregorio Marañon Maternity and Paediatric Hospital in Madrid. Drawn by Victor Carrillo and Daniel Rios, 2021.	110
4.7	A corridor at the Gregorio Marañon Maternity and Paediatric Hospital. Copyright Michael Moran/OTTO.	111
4.8	A patient room at the Gregorio Marañon Maternity and Paediatric Hospital overlooks the corridor. Copyright Michael Moran/OTTO.	113
4.9	Corridor systems project mixed signals about how to be. Drawn by Victor Carrillo and Daniel Rios, 2021.	114
4.10	A chart for building profiles of building users. Image courtesy of Frost Collective.	119
4.11	Northern Beaches Hospital level directories located at key nodal points. Copyright: Toby Peet.	121
4.12	Northern Beaches Hospital atrium graphic. Copyright: Toby Peet.	122
4.13	Original photography created for the environmental graphics. Copyright: Tim Jones.	123
5.1	Floorplan of the Huoshenshan mobile hospital in Wuhan, erected in 2020. Plan redrawn by Victor Carrillo and Daniel Rios, 2021.	134
5.2	The ward with separate circulation loops for nurses and patients at the Huoshenshan hospital. Plan redrawn by Victor Carrillo and Daniel Rios, 2021.	135
5.3	Suspected cases are isolated, while confirmed cases are cohorted. Plan redrawn by Victor Carrillo and Daniel Rios, 2021.	135
5.4	A Fangcang shelter hospital erected in the Wuhan Sports Centre. Copyright: Wang Jing.	136

5.5 NHS Nightingale hospital designed by BDP. Image courtesy of BDP. 138
5.6 Layout, kit out and ventilation principles from the NHS Nightingale manual. Image courtesy of BDP. 139

List of Contributors

Sonit Bafna is an associate professor in the School of Architecture at Georgia Tech, and the director of its PhD program. He works in architectural morphology, addressing problems in interpretation, aesthetics and design theory and developing analytical descriptions of building layouts to explain behavioural patterns and health outcomes. He is currently at work on a book titled 'Imaginative Reasoning in Architecture'.

Jeri Brittin is director of research at HDR. She is a public health research scientist with a background in design and business who works to bring together science and design. She leads HDR's global team of social and behavioural scientists in planning, conducting, publishing and applying research on the built environment and human experience and outcomes. Her research addresses a range of place types, including learning environments, workplaces, health and behavioural facilities and urban and rural communities. She is an active speaker and has published work in numerous journals.

Carlo Giannasca is a multi-award-winning graphic and three-dimensional environmental designer who focuses on wayfinding design and strategy. He embraces complex projects that require a deep and careful assessment of user experience, accessibility and visual communication. Over the past four decades he has created major environmental graphics and wayfinding schemes for projects across a broad range of industry sectors, including health, education and commercial, and is a chapter co-chair of the Society of Experiential Graphic Designers.

Upali Nanda is director of research and a principal with HKS Architects and faculty member at the University of Michigan Taubman School of Architecture and Urban Planning. She leads the research team at HKS and is the executive director of the Center for Advanced Design Research and Evaluation (CADRE), the research arm of HKS. Her work focuses on health and human perception and has been published both in popular and peer-reviewed venues.

Michelle Ossmann is the director of healthcare knowledge and insights for Herman Miller, where she directs health-environment design research and strategy, leads the interior design team and supports product development. She brings over 20 years of clinical and research experience to the relationship between the environment and patient, provider and organisational outcomes. Dr Ossmann is a frequent presenter at design conferences, serves in advisory capacity for various health systems and academic programs and regularly conducts peer reviews for multiple journals.

Rosica Pachilova is an architect by training and recently finished her PhD at University College London in 2020, where she investigated how hospital ward layouts influenced work processes and communication patterns among healthcare providers and how this affected the quality of care provided to patients. Together with Dr Sailer, she won the RIBA President Award for Research in 2019 in the annual theme 'Building in Quality'.

Kerstin Sailer is professor in the sociology of architecture at the Bartlett School of Architecture, University College London. She investigates the impact of spatial design on people and social behaviours inside a range of buildings such as offices, laboratories, hospitals and schools. An architect by training, her research interests combine complex buildings, workplace environments and space usage with social networks, organisational theory and organisational behaviour. She has published widely, and her research has been funded by both industry and various research councils.

George Tingwald uses his combination of qualifications as both an architect and physician in his role as director of medical planning for Stanford Healthcare in Palo Alto, California. The recently opened New Stanford Hospital is the culmination of 15 years of planning, design and construction for Project Renewal for the medical campus. He has served of the Facilities Guidelines Institute for over 25 years and is a founding member of the American College of Healthcare Architects. An accomplished public speaker, Dr. Tingwald is the 2020 recipient of the Changemaker award from the Center for Health Design.

Julie Zook is assistant professor in the College of Architecture at Texas Tech University. Her research focuses on developing typological and morphological models aimed at gaining insights on society and architectural space.

Foreword

Jeri Brittin, PhD

After the House of Commons was destroyed during World War Two, Churchill, in his 28 October 1943 speech to the House of Lords, argued for its reconstruction. Including an oft-repeated extract, his words based on Parliament records follow:

> On the night of 10th May, 1941, with one of the last bombs of the last serious raid, our House of Commons was destroyed by the violence of the enemy, and we have now to consider whether we should build it up again, and how, and when. We shape our buildings and afterwards our buildings shape us. Having dwelt and served for more than 40 years in the late Chamber, and having derived fiery great pleasure and advantage therefrom, I, naturally, would like to see it restored in all essentials to its old form, convenience, and dignity.[1]

A decade later, American philosopher Susanne K. Langer wrote about the 'biological rather than mechanical' notions, including concepts of organic growth and structure, in the work of renowned architects including Sullivan, Wright and Le Corbusier. Langer shed light on a somewhat mysterious human-building inter-relationship – the 'fiery great pleasure and advantage' from a building – that Churchill articulated but had not explained well:

> Because we are organisms, all our actions develop in organic fashion, and our feelings as well as our physical acts have an essentially metabolic pattern. Systole, diastole; making, unmaking, crescendo,

diminuendo. Sustaining, sometimes, but never for indefinite lengths; life, death. Similarly, the human environment, which is the counterpart of any human life, holds the imprint of a functional pattern; it is the complementary organic form. Therefore any building that can create the illusion of an ethnic world, a 'place' articulated by the imprint of human life, must seem organic, like a living form.[2]

In his 1951 treatise, social psychologist Kurt Lewin proposed the notion of 'life space' as a complex field in which individuals and groups act and experience life at given times.[3] Other seminal theoretical work in the social sciences regarding human-environment relations flourished from the 1960s to the 1980s and included the following, among others: Roger Barker proposed the concept of ecological psychology as a means to study and understand environments of human behaviour;[4] William H. Ittelson explained human experience and behaviour as a cognitive synthesis of intended activities, external environmental information and internal information including pre-defined cognitive schemas;[5] Urie Bronfenbrenner's ecology of human development posited 'mutual accommodation throughout the life span' between human organisms and several systemic levels of environmental context, from micro to macro;[6] Harold Proshansky identified the dynamic of place-identity, that our very identities as human beings are intertwined with social-environmental aspects of the settings that we inhabit.[7] And, importantly, building on established social science foundations, architectural scholars Bill Hillier and Julienne Hanson published *The Social Logic of Space* in 1984, a formidable and groundbreaking volume addressing the inextricable linkage of the social and the spatial among human beings. The proposal ran counter to a belief that they thought to be prevalent among architects of the time. The authors called this belief the 'man-environment paradigm': a presumption that environments are merely physical material with no social content and that societies are abstract with no spatial content. Hillier and Hanson posited, quite the contrary, that space is intrinsically social, and that social life is intrinsically spatial.[8] We'll come back to this book shortly.

In 1991, architectural theorist Jon Lang argued that the architecture discipline was primarily focused on creating high art, with emphasis on formalism, and that it should pay more attention to 'the actual behaviors a building is to house'. He went on to explain:

> The two streams of design thought – design as art and design as environmental design – can and should be brought together within

what might tentatively be called a neomodernist normative design theory. It might also be called a behavior deterministic theory because it assumes that design for human behavior, in its multiplicity of complexities, is the purpose of design.[9]

Although Lang's proposal may not have been wholly accepted in the field, substantial interest in understanding and applying hypothesised human-environment relationships was percolating. Healthcare architects, in particular, were attentive to ways that a hospital's design might affect patient comfort and healing. In 1984, Ulrich had published a seminal two-page retrospective medical-records analysis showing that, among patients recovering from gall bladder surgery in one hospital, those with a window facing trees with foliage spent less time hospitalised and needed less pain medication than those with a window facing a brick wall.[10] From the 1990s, healthcare organisations began to adopt evidence-based medicine, which applies evidence from population-based, large controlled trials to inform medical decision making with the goal of improved and more consistent patient outcomes. Inspired by this movement, leading healthcare architects defined 'evidence-based design' as an analogous application of research-generated evidence and best practice in designing healthcare environments focused on improving human outcomes.

Despite the laudable goals and efforts of practising and academic architects and professionals from other disciplines who have been champions of evidence-based design, the field is still very young, and real scientific progress has been slow since the 1990s. Many studies have been published, with authentic intentions among the study designers and authors to create knowledge to improve healthcare environments towards better outcomes for patients and others who occupy these critically important buildings. At the same time, some latched on to claims about 'evidence'-based design as a tactic to sell their services and differentiate themselves from their architectural design competitors. Inadequate research techniques led to simplistic claims of causal connections between specific design features and human outcomes that were desirable to healthcare organisation clients, such as reducing adverse patient events (e.g., infections and falls) and decreasing length of stay. Fortunately, the field is seeing progress, as some of these claims are being addressed in systematic reviews with evidence quality assessments. For example, such recent reviews have found that while single-patient rooms may indeed be more advantageous than disadvantageous overall,[11] there is no convincing evidence for or against providing decentralised stations for caregivers, and no quality empirical evidence demonstrating that presence of decentralised stations leads to reduced patient length of stay.[12]

As Upali Nanda points out in her response to Chapter 3, research questions in the field have not always been well formulated. Where is the cohesive theoretical grounding related to human-environment relationships that exists in the social sciences? Where are plausible models of variable pathway relationships that can be found in the biomedical and public health sciences? Why hasn't there been serious follow-up to Ulrich's seminal 1984 study to see if findings replicate or generalise to larger or more diverse populations? Or to build upon Ulrich's work to identify specific environmental mechanisms beyond what has become known generically as 'views of nature' – aspects of the space, amounts or types of light, visual patterns that stimulate the brain in some way – that may have played some role in the desirable patient outcomes? Even more critical to the future of our field: How might we begin to develop and formalise an ontology for understanding and studying human–built environment relations? Such an ontology – a formalised structure of knowledge, classes, properties and relationships – is vital for scientific progress, and there is much to be learned from examples such as the Ontology for Exposure Science (ExO).[13]

Now, let us come back to the Hillier and Hanson book. Here we have strong theoretical grounding in the social sciences, deep knowledge and practice in the realm of designing architectural space, an understanding that space and society are linked and vary across cultures, and foundations for approaches to construct and measure the social aspects of space quantitatively. While space is three-dimensional and, arguably, the social dynamics of space – the notion of space as complementary to our human selves and activities – must logically occur in three dimensions, healthcare planning often focuses on functionalities in two-dimensional space, with common measures including square-area (square feet or metres) benchmarks such as gross department area per key planning unit (KPU), where an example of a KPU is the patient room.

The 'soft and personal' dimension of hospital architecture noted by Julie Zook in Chapter 1 may indeed be found in the third dimension of what we might call 'human space'. Michelle Ossmann's proposal in Chapter 2 of the importance of the construct 'concurrent visibility' to support effective clinical surveillance makes perfect sense in this context, and George Tingwald's response conveys his related personal experiences. In Chapter 3, Rosi Pachilova and Kerstin Sailer address concepts of community, collaboration and communication in relationship to space and the environment, from Nightingale's pioneering observations of ambient environment influences on patient healing to today; they then introduce the Spaces for Communications Index as an approach to spatial evaluation. Zook and Sonit Bafna address designing for the hospital visitor experience though perceptual and spatial aspects of corridor systems and wayfinding in Chapter 4, with a response from Carlo Giannasca recommending considerable integration of users in a human-centred design process. Sailer proposes (re)inventing 'relational hospitals' based on learning from the pandemic, incorporating constructs such as intelligibility and consideration of the complexities of definitions and inter-relationships of users in Chapter 5. Throughout the book, proposals, ideas and outputs of research are followed by responses from practitioners based on their personal and professional experiences, rendering this work a substantial piece of science that is accessible to all.

We are at a critical time in the field of healthcare architecture, as hospitals have strained and flexed through the recent and current viral pandemic, and we have before us real and tangible opportunities for productive scientific and built innovations in the field of evidence-based design. This volume is timely in addressing critical shifts in thinking and approaches to understand and create embodiments of the social aspects of hospital space in a more cohesive, human-orientated way. With a fiery great pleasure of curiosity, let us proceed to uncover and explore the covert human–spatial life of hospital architecture.

Notes

1 UK Parliament, Hansard 1803–2005, House of Commons Rebuilding, 28 October 1943, vol. 393, cc403-73, https://api.parliament.uk/historic-hansard/commons/1943/oct/28/house-of-commons-rebuilding#S5CV0393P0_19431028_HOC_283 (accessed 20 August 2021).
2 Susanne K. Langer, *Feeling and Form* (New York: Charles Scribner's Sons, 1953), 99.
3 Kurt Lewin, *Field Theory in Social Science* (New York: Harper & Brothers, 1951).
4 Roger G. Barker, *Ecological Psychology: Concepts and Methods for Studying the Environment of Human Behavior* (Redwood City CA: Stanford University Press, 1968).
5 William H. Ittelson, *Environment and Cognition* (Princeton NJ: Seminar Press, 1973).
6 Urie Bronfenbrenner, 'Toward an experimental ecology of human development', *American Psychologist*, 32 (1977), 513–31.
7 Harold Proshansky, 'The city and self-identity', *Environment & Behavior*, 10 (1978), 147–83.
8 Bill Hillier and Julienne Hanson, *The Social Logic of Space* (Cambridge: Cambridge University Press, 1984).
9 Jon Lang, 'Design theory from an environment and behavior perspective', in Erwin H. Zube and Gary T. Moore (eds), *Advances in Environment, Behavior, and Design* (volume 3) (New York: Springer, 1991), 53–101.
10 Roger S. Ulrich, 'View through a window may influence recovery from surgery', *Science*, 224 (1984), 420–1.
11 Ellen Taylor, Alan J. Card and Melissa Piatkowski, 'Single-occupancy patient rooms: a systematic review of the literature since 2006', *Health Environments Research and Design Journal*, 11 (2018), 85–100.

12 Francesqca E. Jimenez, Susan Puumala, Michael Apple, Lou Ann Bunker-Hellmich, Renae K. Rich and Jeri Brittin, 'Associations of patient and staff outcomes with inpatient unit designs incorporating decentralized caregiver workstations: a systematic review of empirical evidence', *Health Environments Research and Design Journal*, 12 (2019), 26–43.

13 Carolyn Mattingly, Thomas McKone, Michael Callahan, Judith Blake and Elaine Cohen Hubal, *Nature Proceedings* (2011) https://doi.org/10.1038/npre.2011.6321.1.

Chapter 1
The spatial dimension of hospital life

Julie Zook

Within the intense functional concerns of hospital architecture, there lurks a soft and personal dimension. Hospital space is experienced by users who are both positioned socially in roles, such as patient, doctor or nurse, and positioned physically in specific locations within a spatial pattern. This book demonstrates ways that the experiential side of hospital architecture systematically and probabilistically affects outcomes. Specifically, this book presents cases where hospital plans are spatially analysed to reveal underlying patterns of paths and visual fields that impact behaviours and outcomes that are important: namely intensive care unit (ICU) mortality, inpatient provider teamwork and hospital wayfinding.

The authors here are interested in how building spaces organise life activities and how built forms are designed to fortify some activities and relationships and not others. For example, built forms convey expectations that nurses are to restore themselves in the break room, escort patients in the hallways and exchange information with other care providers at the designated team station. But in practice, unexpected spatial behaviours and relationships emerge; nurses track doctors in the hallways, talk with patient companions at the station and don't take breaks at all. What a building is made for and what it is used for inevitably fail to fully match up. A building's sanctioned activities are augmented or undermined by informal, emergent ones.[1]

Studying hospital architecture compels attention to the complex social and functional life of buildings. Hospitals present a concentrated version of the challenges that prevail more broadly in architectural thought and practice. An expensive architecture that rarely produces artistic innovation, hospital architecture nevertheless struggles to cope with persistent and sometimes paradoxical functional problems, such as providing patient privacy while maintaining visibility or constraining caregiver travel distances while increasing the size and complexity of hospitals. What is more, the design of hospitals touches on the urgent. Going into the hospital is too often a needlessly harmful or fatal event.[2]

Many rich, industrialised parts of the world are presently in a moment characterised by the imprint of medicine on daily life, a consumerist orientation to health care, access and quality as political issues, looming shortages of healthcare workers and a stratospheric (and climbing) amount of healthcare data that is largely untouched by healthcare architects. These themes are intensified by a global pandemic, escalating climate change and intransigent health inequities. We are challenged to rethink the relationship between society and health, as well as the place of architecture in that relationship.

Architects, for their part, are at long last questioning whether prizing formal novelty has led us too far from professional ideals of social responsibility,[3] whether we are ready to seriously challenge exclusionary practices in the profession[4] and why we have shamefully achieved so little in the face of the climate crisis.[5] It is from this location, this specific tangle of architecture, society and health, that this book was written.

The spatial dimension

The main insights in this book reveal points of contact between the planned and emergent functions of hospitals, with special attention to the moments where the planned and the emergent collide in such a way that they produce outcomes of greater patient safety, increased scope for care-provider communication and more intelligible corridor systems. These phenomena become apparent through forms of spatial analysis that are tied back to tendencies in human spatial perception and cognition, and they probe the question of how spontaneous activities in space – which can be as minute as catching a colleague's eye or reading a patient's facial expression – support the dedicated and planned functions of hospitals. Embedding the user and experience in the measures themselves enables these approaches to sidestep the form-function dichotomy and point in the direction of intentional spatial design.[6]

Social scientists have long recognised the ways that space and society construct and reinforce one another are bound up with how opportunities to use space are afforded to or withheld from individuals and groups.[7] This volume uses approaches from space syntax,[8] which takes as its premise that society and space are mutually constructive and extends this premise into methods for understanding the morphology of buildings plans and city street networks. Space syntax elaborates theorisations of the intrinsic association between society and space by defining spaces mainly in terms of their relationships to one another. One purpose of evaluating spatial configuration is to better describe how space-as-reflecting-society has a patterned relationship to behaviour-as-observed. Another use of space syntax that is especially germane to this book is that syntax-based approaches can give designers insights into how what exists now can form a basis for productively imagining what is possible in the future. There is no shortage of books and research articles on how to design healthcare spaces using evidence. However, too many of these sources are missing clear theoretical foundations that both link to useable measures and provide meaningful explanations of how things work. Explanation in healthcare design research is often based on discrete, individual-level experiences, preferences and outcomes related to building features that are already generally understood to be positive: nature views, privacy, paths free of trip hazards and other broadly beneficial things that are, to be clear, well worth striving for. Absent theory that explains more deeply, data can be collected and calculated in controlled ways, and it can be marshalled to persuade building owners and developers to do better by their buildings' occupants. But this approach to design research runs the risk of too strongly endorsing present conditions, while offering too little with which to transform architecture as a social structure.[9]

Space syntax methods often address the relational properties of the spaces represented in floorplans. In many cases, space syntax measures have predicted human spatial behaviour, with a fairly consistent capacity for relational spatial measures to predict how densities of people are distributed throughout built space. Space syntax is good at revealing how copresence is spatialised.[10] Space syntax can make visible how, under the banner of function or architectural type, profoundly social and affective dimensions of space are quietly installed and enshrined, creating a covert life that arises from ways that floorplan layouts give rise to patterns of visibility, encounter and awareness. This focus on deep, non-obvious and sociologically inflected dimensions of architecture means that space syntax can act as a representational language for insights on how architecture structures social life.[11]

Research, hospitals and architecture

David Theodore describes mid-century architectural research on hospitals in the United Kingdom as modelled on how medicine as a profession integrated scientific research.[12] *The Nuffield Provincial Hospitals Trust Studies in the Functions and Design of Hospitals* investigated design using rational and empirical methods through the 1950s.[13] Two decades later, the *Yale Studies in Hospital Function and Design* undertook a similar task. As their titles suggest, both studies were premised on the importance of establishing a science that identified associations between function and design, with the aim of developing standards for hospital. Both responded to glaring deficits in the post-World-War-II hospital stock. John Thompson and Grace Goldin, of the Yale study, note that what became apparent post-war was that 'the architects did not know how to build hospitals'.[14] They were referring to things like a prevalence of two-foot-wide doors that would make evacuation of bedbound patients impossible in case of fire.

Both studies are remarkable for the range of topics they cover. In Nuffield, these included studies of departments, of caseloads as related to population and of the physical environment, from ventilation to noise and to colour, among other things. Sensibilities and measures from the Nuffield approaches remain with contemporary architectural practice, including the measure square feet per patient bed, nurse-to-patient-to-space ratios and the application of time-motion study techniques to nurse work. Yale, similarly, made broad studies, which included privacy, health-promoting environments, staff supervision and layout efficiency. Regarding layout efficiency, the authors employed the Yale Traffic Index, which aimed at minimising nurse walking distance based on a generalised model of trip frequency and trip length in inpatient units (this study is revisited by Rosica Pachilova and Kerstin Sailer in Chapter 3). Nuffield and Yale call for contemporary hospital design standards through research, with architects as the intended audience of research products.

Both the Yale and Nuffield studies directly correlate design and function. They do not aim to provide insights into individuals or social entities as such or to systematically theorise relations of design to hospital function. There is no attempt to open the black box of causality. There is, instead, the articulation of purely empirical relationships, established through observation and numerical description.

Evidence-based design is a continuation of the kinds of work found in the Nuffield and Yale studies. It tends to emphasise associational links – famously, for example, that nature views speed healing – but invests less in gaining insights about what makes these links work. Sometimes the de-emphasis on theory-building takes the form of the dormitive virtue, a circular logic in which the theory offered for a correlation is just restatement of the correlation in somewhat more abstract or grandiose terms.

Neither the Yale and Nuffield studies nor current approaches in evidence-based design invest in the development of the sorts of theory that answer *why* two things are associated. The missing explanation of the why means that studies can point to specific solutions to narrowly defined problems, but they cannot supply designers with principles that let them approach problems flexibly and creatively, as designers tend to do.

The main chapters in this book actively seek explanations by creating theories of the social function of hospital spaces. Instead of just looking for empirical associations, they push back on assumptions embedded in existing measures, through either direct critique or the development of new measures with clearly stated areas of interest in human experience, cognition and behaviour.

Sonit Bafna has noted the general tendency of architectural designers to employ tangible, visual forms when they are trying to effect sociological change.[15] This book takes a different approach by focusing on spatial form as revealed in floorplans, a latent aspect of design that reflects sociological dimensions of architecture. Certain healthcare problems find their realisation in space, and hospital and healthcare architects seem generally aware of the central importance of the plan in grappling with these dilemmas.[16]

Space – continuous, flowing and often invisible to the mind's eye – would seem to naturally resist analysis, and, indeed, finding ways to chunk inhabitable space into individual-but-connected units is, all by itself, an analytical act. A key concept in space syntax is that patterns of spatial depth can be used to calculate segregation or integration values for spaces. Space syntax metrics, such as integration values, make it possible to describe space in precise and reliable ways that can be entered into statistical models together with data on outcomes or observed behaviours.[17]

Space syntax theories about society and space were initially developed throughout the 1970s. In subsequent decades, syntax measures were tested against observed behaviour in empirical studies in urban areas, then in other settings, including offices, museums and hospitals.[18] In practice, much of the behaviourally orientated syntax research proceeds by associating dimensions of layout with how building users are observed to engage with space and with people and things in space.

Syntax studies on behaviour have inferred a great deal from distributions of people in space in particular, following the Goffmanian notion of copresence as presenting latent resources.[19] Space syntax as a field could do more to unpack how copresence works and understand what people experience and do in space in greater detail, particularly in settings like hospitals. Several approaches in the book aim at more detailed insight on spatial experience and behaviour as linked to floorplan morphology.

Ivan Illich blasted the 'medicalization of life' in his 1975 essay outlining ways that medicine has increased its extents, giving us greater opportunity to monitor and control our corporeal selves, but at significant psychological and economic costs.[20] The possibility implicit in this volume is that it is both conceivable and necessary to rethink the function of healthcare spaces so that they might do more justice to who we are, to our keenness to experience and to understand and be understood and to the importance that we place on associations and on the exercise of our creative capabilities.

New forms of healthcare architecture

A difficulty of discussing, let alone realising, such humanistic aspirations for healthcare spaces is that their conceptual categories are not necessarily congruent with architectural ones. One way to approach the gap is from its two poles: the architectural type and the behaviour setting. These two concepts correspond to idealised and empirical approaches to design.

Architectural types are generally thought of both in terms of forms that recur (e.g., pavilion, plinth or tower) as well as in terms of culturally agreed upon functions (e.g., hospital, prison or school).[21] Types consist of morphological forms related to functions. They are understood as abstract entities that provide organisational principles and can be transformed and concretised in innumerable ways based on specific exigencies. J. N. L. Durand linked architecture to society through architectural types in their capacity to give form to programme, a conception still current in at least some accounts.[22] But types are also social insofar as they are created with the imaginative projection of some codified form of life in mind, some expected stereotypical patterns of activity.

Rafael Moneo has referred to the emergence of new building types as one of 'the most intense moments in architectural development'.[23] But new types seem to come less often from our most brilliant architects than from clients, public and private, who, as part of their daily lives, see the

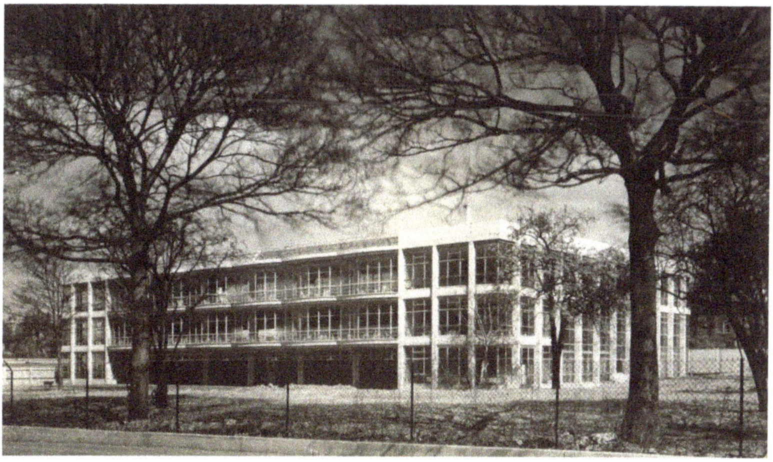

1.1 The transparent architecture of the Pioneer Health Centre, 1935 Dell & Wainwright/RIBA Collections.

gaps between what architectural types supply and the actual activities that require accommodation.

'Behaviour settings', a concept from environmental psychology, are useful for understanding how behaviour is shaped by its ecological context: that is, by being a part of some socially instituted activity. Behaviour settings are patterns of standing behaviour that develop in environments shaped to facilitate them, so the concept of the behaviour setting acts as a fundamental unit for studying the relationship of behaviour and space.[24] For example, hosting a dinner party entails a set of spaces, people and objects that are ordered to some degree so that the 'dinner party' activity can take place. Recent scholarship has extended perspectives on behaviour settings to address how they originate, respond to contexts and shape sense-making.[25]

The main reason for using behaviour settings is to determine the fundamental unit at which behaviour makes sense and can be explained and tied to space. They provide a basis for discretisation of activity and of space. Human activity can be viewed as a matter of participation in successive behaviour settings, and a building can be thought of as a collection of specific behaviour settings that are brought together either because they organically relate to each other or so that they can share physical resources. Because behaviour settings occur in clumps, set ways of organising them into groups result in architectural types.

In the two cases described here – a London-based health centre and a Phoenix-based ambulatory surgical centre – clients created new

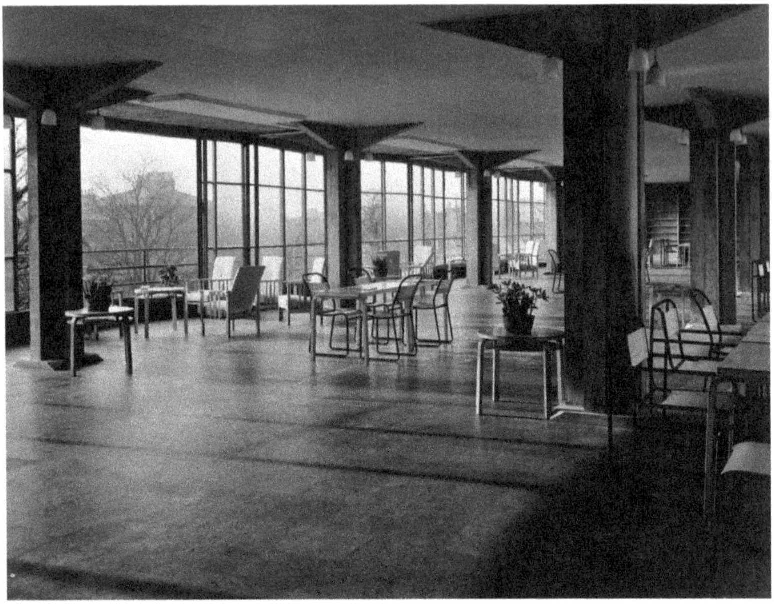

1.2 Unpartitioned space at the Pioneer Health Centre, Dell & Wainwright/RIBA Collections.

activities that required new behaviour settings to be organised into new architectural types. These two very different instances demonstrate ways that behaviour setting and architectural form interact when a type is born.

In 1935, the Pioneer Health Centre opened in South London as part of the Peckham Experiment, which aimed to establish 'ethology', a newly invented field that intended to focus on health, as distinct from the treatment of illness. The Pioneer Health Centre was established by two biologist physicians who advocated ethology, spouses Dr George Scott Williamson and Dr Innes H. Pearse. The building itself was designed by celebrated architectural engineer Sir Owen Williams as three reinforced-concrete slabs on a column grid with an atrium pool at the centre. The façade was almost fully glazed (see Figure 1.1) and much of the interior was intervisible (see Figure 1.2). The transparency of the building existed to allow surveillance by the doctors, but it was also said to embed an aesthetic of human activity that encouraged participation in the Centre's activities. The building included double-height lecture and gym spaces (see Figure 1.3), one-storey spaces for play and lounging (see Figure 1.4) and, tucked away on the highest level, rooms for medical examination. In the clinic spaces, patients were examined, but not treated, in exclusive

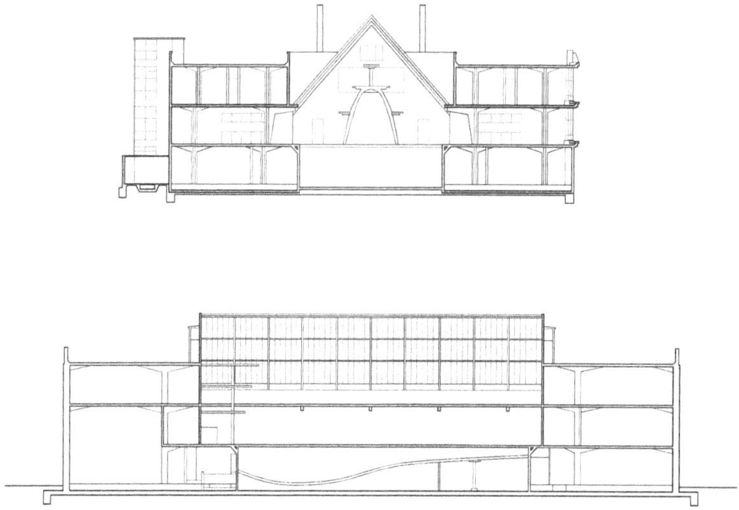

1.3 Pioneer Health Centre sections, as drawn by Victor Carrillo and Daniel Rios, 2021.

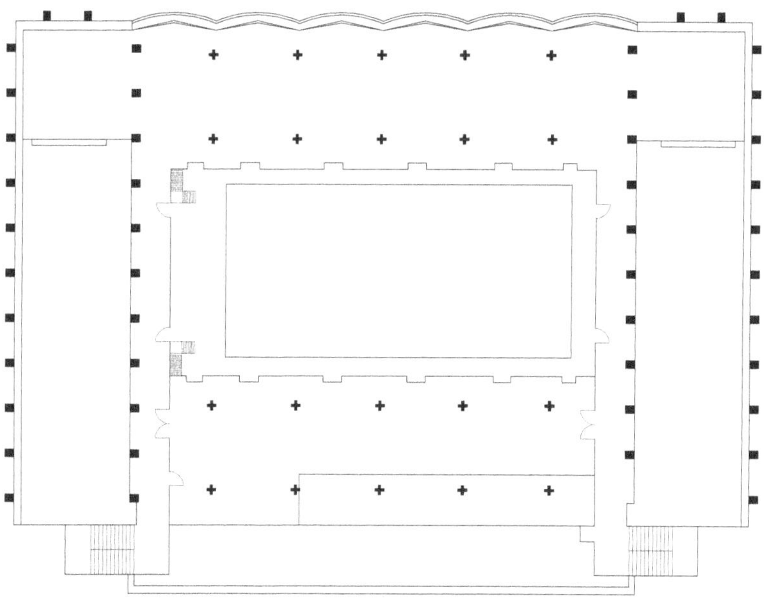

1.4 Pioneer Health Centre floorplan, as drawn by Victor Carrillo and Daniel Rios, 2021. The first floor (one level above ground) has lounge and cafeteria spaces on the long arms of the plan, overlooks to recreation spaces on the short arms, and the pool at the centre.

focus on discovering the principles of health. Patients had to be referred out if they wanted medical treatment. Outside of the clinic, the everyday functioning of the Pioneer Health Centre was organised by its members. Membership was restricted to neighbourhood residents, and they were required to join as family units, not as individuals.

The Peckham Experiment promoted the ideals and practices of positive health, regular check-ups, the family as the unit of intervention and the social field as relevant to health. The building was accordingly open, flexible and programmed for self-directed and spontaneous activity. While its doctors seemed to anticipate epidemiology in some ways, other dimensions of the Peckham Experiment were regressive. It extended the medical gaze to recreation, it enforced a specific form of family life and it aimed at so-called 'positive' eugenics. The doctors collected data on health that included tabulations of 'suitable-mate' marriages and births that had taken place under the influence of the health centre, publishing in journals such as *The Eugenics Review*.[26] Even when not focused on breeding an improved human, Peckham's science tended to emphasise normative ideas about health and 'right living' advanced by methodologically weak science.[27]

The Pioneer Health Centre was shuttered in 1950. It could not maintain funding through the combination of gifts and membership dues on which it had subsisted, and it failed to find a place either as part of the newly formed National Health Service[28] or as a research organisation. The building stands today as part of a gated residential community – its radically open plan is subdivided, its spaces for spontaneous social activity renovated into apartments.

In 1970, 20 years after the Pioneer Health Centre closed, the first freestanding ambulatory surgical centre in the United States opened in Phoenix, Arizona. Dr Wallace Reed and Dr John Ford had opened their 'Surgicenter' after years of planning and coordination with government bodies, insurers and healthcare groups. Five physicians performed five surgeries that day, including four using general anaesthesia.

At the time the new type was initiated, ambulatory surgeries were being performed in emergency departments. Not only was this arrangement expensive, but surgeries would be delayed in the entirely probable event of an emergency patient requiring the room. In the retelling of the development of a new building type, though, a surprisingly pedestrian and relatable agenda was among the initiating forces: that of strategising to manage personal exhaustion. According to Dr Reed:

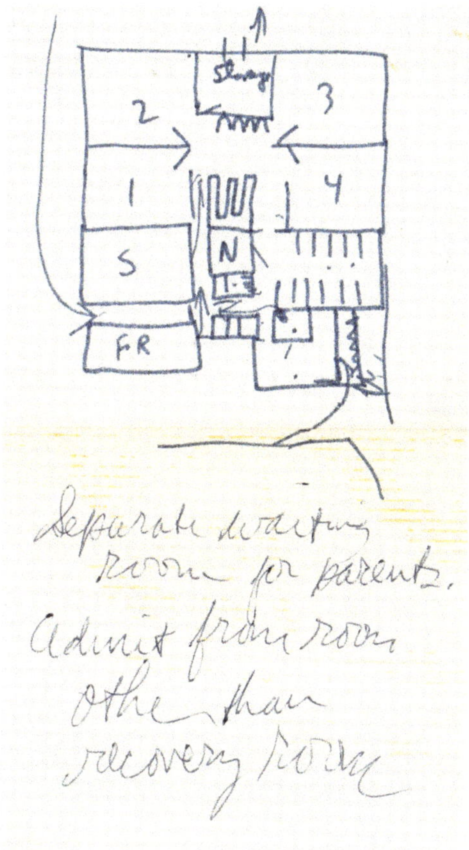

1.5 Dr Reed's sketch plan of Surgicenter, Wood Library, Museum of Anesthesiology.

> [Dr] Jack [Ford] and I were in mid-career. I was in my 50s, and he was close to it, and we were thinking about how we were going to extend our careers. We knew we weren't going to be able to continue doing cases all night and then taking on a regular schedule during the day.[29]

Dr Reed and Dr Ford saw the exhaustion, lost time and unnecessary expense as infringements on patients and providers that were a part of a context of well-recognised inadequacies in outpatient care. Their idea for a freestanding surgery building was aimed at providing reliable scheduling, high-care quality, insurance reimbursement and a good environment for providers and patients.

Ambulatory surgery consists of a tightly choreographed sequence of predictable activities: from intake to pre-operative care, to surgery and recovery. Dr Reed literally sketched out a bare-bones scheme to accommodate these activities, plus auxiliary activities such as waiting and records, in a plan of about 5,000 square feet that emphasised a circular patient flow (see Figure 1.5).

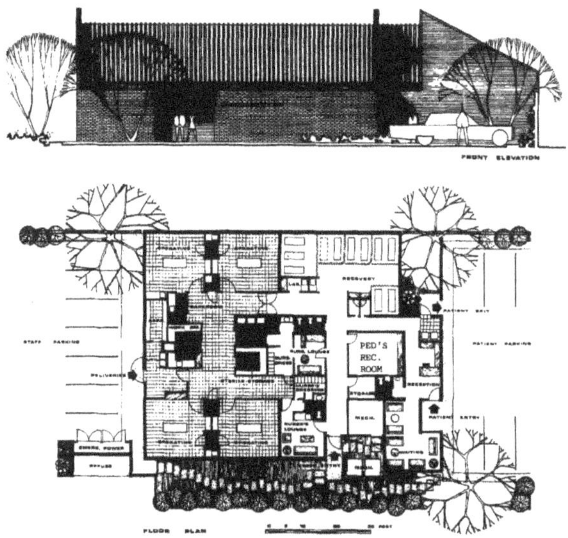

1.6 The Surgicenter floorplan and elevation, reprinted from the *Journal of Pediatric Surgery*, Vol. 7, Daniel T. Cloud, Wallace A. Reed, John L. Ford, Laurence M. Linkner, David S. Trump and George W. Dorman, 'The surgicenter: A fresh concept in outpatient pediatric surgery' (1972), 207, with permission from Elsevier.

Working with an architect whose name is not disclosed in the project publicity and scholarly accounts,[30] the 'Surgicenter' was developed as a highly successful new type that would go on to be repeated thousands of times and house millions of procedures. The original Surgicenter building itself was modest, but of some presence: a brick exterior with a single-pitch metal roof and deeply recessed window and entrance openings. Though sparse, it managed to evince an off-type styling that responded to trends of its time, perhaps in keeping with its orientation to the concerns and experiences of individual care providers and patients (see Figure 1.6). In a write up of the 'handsome, one-story building' in the *Association of periOperative Registered Nurses Journal*, the author, a registered nurse, is impressed with 'the warm shades of stained wood against the exposed brick' and 'the thick, burnt orange carpeting'.[31]

What ambulatory surgical centres gave surgeons, staff and patients was a set of rationally linked behaviour settings that cohered around the outpatient surgery and its associated activities, held together in a new building type. The real labour of implementing the type was less in conceiving of and specifying the design of the facility – which seems to have emerged all but spontaneously and fully formed – than in persuading an array of insurers, health maintenance organisations and state and national governing bodies to permit surgeries to proceed and be reimbursed. In the early 1990s, the original Surgicenter moved to a new location in Phoenix. The practice needed more space, and the existing building no longer came up to the code requirements that it had helped establish.

I have described two new healthcare building types from the twentieth century, each resting on a client proposal for new routines in medical space. The Pioneer Health Centre implemented as a type the intervisible and transparent box that propagates the social field as a locus of wellness. By contrast, ambulatory surgical centres cohered around the highly predictable flow of outpatient surgery, newly emplaced in a building of its own.

In his book, *Building Types and Built Forms*, Phil Steadman outlines potential reasons for the demise of building types, including competition between activities and between the built forms that accommodate these activities.[32] The Pioneer Health Centre appears to have fared poorly in competition with the services offered by the newly formed National Health Service, while the Surgicenter type provided a much-preferred alternative to emergency department and hospital-based surgery. These two building types also reflect what David Theodore terms 'the decline of the hospital as a healing machine',[33] whereby the hospital (or healthcare) building itself acted less, over time, as the direct agent of healing, as the Pioneer Centre aimed to do, and more as instrument of the rational administration of healthy populations.

These two cases, where entirely new settings were created, focus the discussion of what healthcare architecture does to society and to the finer grain of how society accommodates and organises activities inside a specific instance of an architectural type. Such a focus is relevant in introducing this book because architects work in types – types of buildings, of inpatient units, of nursing stations, of corridor networks. They ask, 'which is best?' for a project or a specific problem. This volume draws attention away from the gross-grain aspects of type to something much finer and closer to the behaviour setting, to something that conveys ways that layouts position our perceptual apparatus and thus selectively reveal the world to us and probabilistically modulate our actions. Many important commitments in the design of hospital architecture take place at this level, with architects not always aware that they have made these commitments until well after the building is constructed and in use, if ever they are aware at all.

Pillow, Table, Hallway

The organisation of the main chapters as 'Pillow', 'Table' and 'Hallway' reflects the aim of the book to spotlight various elements and scales of space that are associated with different roles – namely, patients, care teams and hospital visitors. We have adopted metaphoric labels that both emphasise the multiple scales at which hospitals function and call to mind the familiar things that comprise much of hospital life. The hospital's carceral genealogy notwithstanding,[34] it is the everyday relations in hospital space that are the main focus of this book. Because we are interested in the applicability of the research to the problems of society as addressed through the design professions, we have invited knowledgeable leaders from practice to write essays that respond to each main chapter and bring in their own perspectives.

Michelle Ossmann opens Chapter 2, 'Pillow', with a study of visibility and chart data in ICU environments that demonstrates the life-saving potential of a specific form of visual link between the patient bedhead and the unit at large. Gary Tingwald – doctor, architect and medical planning director – responds with an account of his personal and professional experiences of ICU design. Rosica Pachilova and Kerstin Sailer's chapter, 'Table', develops a visibility index that measures the communication potential for nurses in inpatient wards. Upali Nanda, an industry-based research director, responds with an essay on nurse work concepts applied in architectural practice and the continued need for good measures. In 'Hallway', Sonit Bafna and I investigate the hospital corridor system and the inherent tension between the physical and organisational complexity of hospitals and the visitor's need for navigable and intelligible space, a tension amplified by popular misunderstandings about cognition among designers, as well as by ambivalence towards the hospital as an institution. Environmental graphic designer Carlo Giannasca responds by describing a programme and process for user-centred design. The volume closes with a chapter by Kerstin Sailer that describes responses and conditions of COVID-19 from within the sociological conception of space that characterises this volume, laying out what this conception implies for the definition of 'user' in healthcare architecture.

Our book neglects to address two particularly important areas of hospital design and its relation to society. We do not address hospital energy use or embodied energy, even though hospitals are problematic energy consumers.[35] And although we account thoroughly for some roles in buildings, we do not account for the social locations of individuals and groups and how these locations affect experience and outcomes. Structures of visual connectivity are impartial as to who is in a hospital space, but persistent and well-documented disparities in healthcare by race indicate that the same cannot be said for healthcare systems and workers.[36]

Some readers may be disappointed that this book is primarily analytical, offering no overarching theory for generating good hospital form. This is intentional. It is very easy to declare how some architectural approach will work, but very difficult to capture nuanced but generalisable descriptions of how it actually does work. The volume takes on this latter, less glamorous task because it is foundational to developing theories of building function that can offer a stronger and more flexible basis for design decisions.

Designing, constructing and inhabiting hospitals are endeavours marked by uncertainty and risk. This book presents principles that have been tested empirically. The syntax analysis used involves a reflective approach to quantification that might stimulate new ideas for readers on how to relate data and design. The authors write from a conviction that to deeply understand hospital spaces is to attend to key dimensions that organise life, society and architecture in general, and so the book is intended to be of broad interest to architects and others interested in how we live through built forms. Although we focus little on aesthetics as such, several descriptions address how layout, and other properties of hospitals, shape something like subjectivity in built space.

This book was assembled to convey insights about the non-obvious and non-trivial things that happen in hospital architecture because of design. It focuses on space because space structures our life patterns, framing and conditioning individual and social actions. It uses rigorous methods, not because science provides the proof to finally settle questions, but because careful enquiry stimulates better questions and better formulation of problems. Our intent is to make overt some instances and tactics – glimpses, as it were – that offer models for the organisation of hospital space under a conception of architectural function that might better support human flourishing.

Notes

1 For a discussion of the generative dimension of organisational routines, see Martha S. Feldman and Brian T. Pentland, 'Reconceptualizing organizational routines as a source of flexibility and change', *Administrative Science Quarterly*, 48 (2003), 94–118.

2 The Institute of Medicine landmark report *To Err is Human* identified a shockingly high prevalence of preventable patient harm, including death. Bates and Singh's appraisal of progress since *To Err is Human*, found that preventable patient harms persist at a high rate and that future breakthroughs may depend on mobilising new insights (2018). The Institute of Medicine (US) Committee on Quality of Health Care in America. Linda T. Kohn *et al.* (eds), *To Err is Human: Building a Safer Health System* (Washington DC: National Academies Press, 2000). https://doi.org/10.17226/9728. David W. Bates and Hardeep Singh, 'Two decades since *To Err is Human*: an assessment of progress and emerging priorities in patient safety', *Health Affairs (Project Hope)*, 37, 11 (2018), 1736–43, https://doi.org/10.1377/hlthaff.2018.0738.

3 See, for example, Kate Wagner, 'Coronagrifting: a design phenomenon', https://mcmansionhell.com/post/618938984050147328/coronagrifting-a-design-phenomenon (accessed 3 April 2021).

4 See, for example, Wallace Ludel, 'Artists and architects ask MoMA and other institutions to remove Philip Johnson's name citing his racist views', *The Arts Newspaper* (4 December 2020), https://www.theartnewspaper.com/news/artists-and-architects-ask-moma-and-other-institution-to-remove-philip-johnson-s-name-citing-his-racist-views (accessed 3 April 2021).

5 See, for example, Billy Fleming, 'Design and the Green New Deal', *Places Journal* (April 2019), https://doi.org/10.22269/190416 (accessed 2 April 2021).

6 Though working in a different ontology, a related aspiration is conveyed by Anthony Vidler for new approaches to architectural programming in Anthony Vidler, 'Toward a theory of the architectural program', *October*, 106, Fall (2003), 65.

7 Much of this work comes from feminist and Marxist geography, for example, Doreen Massey, *Space, Place, and Gender* (Minneapolis MN: University of Minnesota Press, 1994); and Edward Soja, *Postmodern Geographies: The Reassertion of Space in Critical Social Theory* (London and New York: Verso, 1989).

8 Space syntax argues that society and space are mutually constructive. In the first major book on space syntax, *The Social Logic of Space*, Bill Hillier and Julienne Hanson set out an extensive programme of research into spatial and social structures, including spatial discretisations and calculations, as well as a number of case studies of an anthropological flavour: Bill Hillier and Julienne Hanson, *The Social Logic of Space* (Cambridge: Cambridge University Press, 1984). Only in subsequent work were the measures found to correlate with behaviours. For a later overview of space syntax, see Sonit Bafna, 'Space syntax: a brief introduction to its logic and techniques', *Environment and Behavior*, 35, 1 (2003), 17–29.

9 Anthony Giddens, *New Rules of Sociological Method* (second edition) (Redwood City CA: Stanford University Press, 1993). For a critique of the lack of institutional imagination, see Roberto M. Unger, *What Should Legal Analysis Become?* (London and New York: Verso, 1995).

10 See, for example, Tadeusz Grajewski, 'The SAS head office: spatial configuration and interaction patterns', *Nordic Journal of Architectural Research*, 2 (1993), 63–74. See also Alan Penn, Justin Desyllas and Laura Vaughan, 'The space of innovation: interaction and communication in the work environment', *Environment and Planning (B): Planning and Design*, 26, (1999), 193–218.

11 Space syntax theory is distinct from architectural theories generally insofar as it is mainly analytical and mainly aimed at producing insights. Many architecture theories – landscape urbanism, for example – are aimed at assisting designers in generating designs according to the principles rendered by the theorist, with the theorist generally prognosticating how the designs will work. Bill Hillier characterises such architectural theory as 'too often ... strongly normative and weakly analytic', the trouble with which is that 'it has been too easy to use [architectural theories] to generate designs, but they are too weak in predicting what these designs will be like when built'. Hillier, *Space is the Machine: A Configurational Theory of Architecture* (Cambridge: Cambridge University Press, 1996), 2.

12 In an article describing the Nuffield Trust, David Theodore outlines the structural correspondence between mid-century architectural research on hospitals in the United Kingdom and medical models for the integration of research into professions. See David Theodore, 'Treating architectural research: the Nuffield Trust and the post-war hospital,' *Journal of Architecture*, 21, 7 (2019), 982–98.

13 Nuffield Provincial Hospitals Trust, *Studies in the Functions and Design of Hospitals* (London: Oxford University Press, 1955).

14 John D. Thompson and Grace Goldin, *The Hospital: A Social and Architectural History* (New Haven CT and London: Yale University Press, 1975), 253.

15 Sonit Bafna, 'The imaginative function of architecture: a clarification of some conceptual issues', in Margarita Greene, José Reyes and Andrea Castro (eds), *Proceedings of the Eighth International Symposium on Space Syntax* (Santiago: Pontificia Universidad Catolica de Chile, 2012), 8117, 1–15.

16 In the early twentieth century, hospital architect Edward F. Stevens declared, 'Unlike most architectural problems, the plan of the hospital is the strongest factor in the design'. Edward F. Stevens, 'The American hospital development, Part I', *Architectural Record*, 38 (December 1915), 645. I first encountered Stevens and his views on hospital architecture in Annmarie Adams, *Medicine by Design: The Architect and the Modern Hospital, 1893–1943* (Minneapolis MN: University of Minnesota Press, 2008), 129.

17 A key step, described only briefly here, is that the space syntax calculations are run atop graph theoretic representations of configured space taken from the initial discretisation. An overview of the theory that emphasises the conceptual importance of depth in space syntax can be found in Bill Hillier and Julienne Hanson, *The Social Logic of Space* (Cambridge: Cambridge University Press, 1984).

18 In addition to being associated with high densities of people, space syntax measures of integration have tended to anchor certain spaces for purposes of orientation. See John Peponis, Craig Zimring and Yoon Kyung Choi, 'Finding the building in wayfinding', *Environment and Behavior*, 22, 5 (1990), 555–90; and Saif Haq and Craig Zimring, 'Just down the road a piece: the development of topological knowledge of building layouts', *Environment and Behavior*, 35, 1 (2003), 132–60.

19 Erving Goffman, *Interaction Ritual: Essays on Face-to-Face Behavior* (Garden City NY: Doubleday, 1967).

20 Ivan Illich, 'Medicalization of life', *Journal of Medical Ethics*, I, 2 (1975), 73–7.

21 Adrian Forty, 'Type', in *Words and Buildings: A Vocabulary of Modern Architecture* (New York: Thames & Hudson, 2004), 304–11; Philip Steadman, *Building Types and Built Forms* (Leicestershire: Matador, 2014).

22 Rafael Moneo, 'On typology', *Oppositions*, 13 [](1978), 23–45. Antoine Picone, 'From "poetry of art" to method: the theory of Jean-Nicolas-Louis Durand', in *Précis des Leçons D'architecture Données à l'École Polytechnique Texts and Documents* (Los Angeles CA: Getty Research Institute, 2001), 1–68. Vidler, *'Toward a theory of the architectural program'*.

23 Moneo, 'On typology', 27.

24 For behaviour settings, see Roger Barker and Paul Gump, *Big School, Small School* (Stanford CA: Stanford University Press, 1964); and Roger Barker and Phil Schoggen, *Qualities of*

Community Life: Methods of Measuring Environment and Behavior Applied to an American and an English Town (San Francisco CA: Jossey-Bass, 1973).

25 For extended perceptions on behaviour settings, see Allan Wicker, 'Perspectives on behavior settings: with illustrations from Allison's ethnography of a Japanese hostess club', *Environment and Behavior*, 44, 4 (2012), 474–92.

26 Mary Gowing, 'Incentives to parenthood: some data from the Pioneer Health Centre, Peckham', *The Eugenics Review*, 35, 2 (1943), 39–41.

27 Philip Conford, '"Smashed by the National Health"? A closer look at the demise of the Pioneer Health Centre, Peckham', *Medical History*, 60, 2 (2016), 250–69.

28 For a recent scholarship on the contemporary National Health Service's health centre type, see Justin De Syllas, *Integrating Care: The Architecture of the Comprehensive Health Centre* (New York: Routledge, 2015).

29 Ambulatory Surgical Center Association, 'Looking back and looking forward from where it all began', *FASA Update* (May/June 2004), https://www.ascassociation.org/communities/community-home/librarydocuments/viewdocument?DocumentKey=8c767384-8a84-4dd7-a729-f423407229cb (accessed 4 April 2021).

30 Dr Philip identifies Dr Reed as the facility designer, showing his original sketch plan for the center in 'Phoenix Surgery Center Design Drawing (Smuggler's Inn Card)' (15 October 2019), https://www.youtube.com/watch?v=Qjeds6CsJ8g&t=1s (accessed 11 April 2021).

31 Audrey Bell, 'Day surgery: a concept of care for the pediatric patient', *AORN*, 19, 3 (1974), 623–31.

32 Philip Steadman, 'Building types and how they change over time', in *Building Types and Built Forms* (Leicestershire: Matador, 2014), 353–84.

33 David Theodore, 'The decline of the hospital as a healing machine', in Sarah Schrank and Didem Ekici (eds), *Healing Spaces, Modern Architecture, and the Body* (New York, Routledge, 2017), 186–203.

34 Thomas Markus, *Buildings and Power: Freedom and Control in the Origin of Modern Building Types* (London: Routledge, 1993).

35 Hospitals have high energy-use intensity. See Luis Pérez-Lombard, José Ortiz and Christine Pout, 'A review on buildings energy consumption information', *Energy and Buildings*, 40, 3 (2008), 394–8.

36 See, for example, Vickie M. Mays, Susan D. Cochran and Namdi W. Barnes, 'Race, race-based discrimination, and health outcomes among African Americans', *Annual Review of Psychology*, 58 (2007), 201–25, https://doi.org/10.1146/annurev.psych.57.102904.190212.

References

Adams, Annmarie, *Medicine by Design: The Architect and the Modern Hospital, 1893–1943* (Minneapolis MN: University of Minnesota Press, 2008).

Ambulatory Surgical Center Association, 'Looking back and looking forward from where it all began', *FASA Update* (May/June 2004) https://www.ascassociation.org/communities/community-home/librarydocuments/viewdocument?DocumentKey=8c767384-8a84-4dd7-a729-f423407229cb.

Bafna, Sonit, 'Space syntax: a brief introduction to its logic and techniques', *Environment and Behavior*, 35, 1 (2003), 17–29.

Bafna, Sonit, 'The imaginative function of architecture: a clarification of some conceptual issues', in Margarita Greene, José Reyes and Andrea Castro (eds), *Proceedings of the Eighth International Symposium on Space Syntax* (Santiago: Pontificia Universidad Catolica de Chile, 2012), 8117, 1 -15.

Barker, Roger, and Paul Gump, *Big School, Small School* (Stanford CA: Stanford University Press, 1964).

Barker, Roger G., and Phil Schoggen, *Qualities of Community Life: Methods of Measuring Environment and Behavior Applied to an American and an English Town* (San Francisco CA: Jossey-Bass, 1973).

Bates, David W., and Hardeep Singh, 'Two decades since *To Err is Human*: an assessment of progress and emerging priorities in patient safety', *Health Affairs (Project Hope)*, 37, 11 (2018), 1736–43, https://doi.org/10.1377/hlthaff.2018.0738.

Bell, Audrey, 'Day surgery: a concept of care for the pediatric patient', *AORN*, 19, 3 (1974), 623–31.
Conford, Philip, '"Smashed by the National Health?" A closer look at the demise of the Pioneer Health Centre, Peckham', *Medical History*, 60, no. 2 (2016), 250–69.
De Syllas, Justin, *Integrating Care: The Architecture of the Comprehensive Health Centre* (New York: Routledge, 2015).
Feldman, Martha S., and Brian T. Pentland, 'Reconceptualizing organizational routines as a source of flexibility and change', *Administrative Science Quarterly*, 48 (2003), 94–118.
Fleming, Billy, 'Design and the Green New Deal', *Places Journal* (April 2019), https://doi.org/10.22269/190416.
Forty, Adrian, 'Type', in *Words and Buildings: A Vocabulary of Modern Architecture* (New York: Thames & Hudson, 2004), 304–11.
Foucault Michel, *The Birth of the Clinic: An Archaeology of Medical Perception* (London: Tavistock, 1973).
Giddens, Anthony, *New Rules of Sociological Method* (second edition) (Redwood City CA: Stanford University Press, 1993).
Goffman, Erving, *Interaction Ritual: Essays on Face-to-Face Behavior* (Garden City NY: Doubleday, 1967).
Gowing, Mary, 'Incentives to parenthood: some data from the Pioneer Health Centre, Peckham', *The Eugenics Review*, 35, 2 (1943), 39–41.
Grajewski, Tadeusz, 'The SAS head office: spatial configuration and interaction patterns', *Nordic Journal of Architectural Research*, 2 (1993), 63–74.
Haq, Saif, and Craig Zimring, 'Just down the road a piece: the development of topological knowledge of building layouts', *Environment and Behavior*, 35, 1 (2003), 132–60.
Hillier, Bill, *Space is the Machine: A Configurational Theory of Architecture* (Cambridge: Cambridge University Press, 1996), https://discovery.ucl.ac.uk/id/eprint/3881/1/SITM.pdf.
Hillier, Bill, and Julienne Hanson, *The Social Logic of Space* (Cambridge: Cambridge University Press, 1984).
Illich, Ivan, 'Medicalization of life', *Journal of Medical Ethics*, I, 2 (1975), 73–7.
Kohn, Linda T., *et al.* (eds), '*To Err is Human: Building a safer health system*', Institute of Medicine (Washington DC: National Academies Press, 2000), https://doi.org/10.17226/9728.
Ludel, Wallace, 'Artists and architects ask MoMA and other institutions to remove Philip Johnson's name citing his racist views', *The Arts Newspaper*, (4 December 2020), https://www.theartnewspaper.com/news/artists-and-architects-ask-moma-and-otherinstitution-to-remove-philip-johnson-s-name-citing-his-racist-views.
Markus, Thomas A., *Buildings and Power: Freedom and Control in the Origin of Modern Building Types* (London: Routledge, 1993).
Massey, Doreen, *Space, Place, and Gender* (Minneapolis MN: University of Minnesota Press, 1994).
Mays, Vickie M., Susan D. Cochran and Namdi W. Barnes, 'Race, race-based discrimination, and health outcomes among African Americans', *Annual Review of Psychology*, 58 (2007), 201–25, https://doi.org/10.1146/annurev.psych.57.102904.190212.
Moneo, Rafael, 'On typology', *Oppositions*, 13 (1978), 23–45.
Peponis, John, Craig Zimring and Yoon Kyung Choi, 'Finding the building in wayfinding', *Environment and Behavior*, 22, 5 (1990), 555–90, https://doi.org/10.1177/0013916590225001.
Pérez-Lombard, Luis, José Ortiz and Christine Pout, 'A review on buildings energy consumption information', *Energy and Buildings*, 40, 3 (2008), 394–8.
Picone, Antoine, 'From "poetry of art" to method: the theory of Jean-Nicolas-Louis Durand', in *Précis des Leçons D'architecture Données à l'École Polytechnique Texts and Documents* (Los Angeles CA: Getty Research Institute, 2001), 1–68.
Soja, Edward, *Postmodern Geographies: The Reassertion of Space in Critical Social Theory* (London and New York: Verso, 1989).
Steadman, Philip, 'Building types and how they change over time', in *Building Types and Built Forms* (Leicestershire: Matador, 2014), 353–84.
Stevens, Edward F., *The American Hospital Development: Part I* (New York: The Architectural Record Company, 1915).
Theodore, David, 'The decline of the hospital as a healing machine', in Sarah Schrank and Didem Ekici (eds), *Healing Spaces, Modern Architecture, and the Body* (New York: Routledge, 2017), 186–202.
Theodore, David, 'Treating architectural research: the Nuffield Trust and the post-war hospital', *Journal of Architecture*, 21, 7 (2019), 982–98.

Thompson, John D., and Grace Goldin, *The Hospital: A Social and Architectural History* (New Haven CT and London: Yale University Press, 1975).
Unger, Roberto M., *What Should Legal Analysis Become?* (London and New York: Verso, 1995).
Vidler, Anthony, 'Toward a theory of the architectural program', *October*, 106, Fall (2003), 59–74.
Wagner, Kate, 'Coronagrifting: a design phenomenon', (2020) https://mcmansionhell.com/post/618938984050147328/coronagrifting-a-design-phenomenon.
Wicker, Allan, 'Perspectives on behavior settings: with illustrations from Allison's ethnography of a Japanese hostess club', *Environment and Behavior*, 44, 4 (2012), 474–92.
Wood Library – Museum of Anesthesiology, 'Phoenix Surgery Center Design Drawing (Smuggler's Inn Card)', YouTube (15 October 2019), https://www.youtube.com/watch?v=Qjeds6CsJ8g&t=1s.

Chapter 2: Pillow
Introduction

In this chapter, Michelle Ossmann presents a novel approach to assessing patient surveillance based on floorplan layout analysis. Similar prior approaches have been based largely on direct line-of-sight visual connections. Ossmann critiques these as failing to embody a full understanding of surveillance, which includes cognitive and behavioural dimensions. Accordingly, her floorplan measure – which emanates from the patient 'pillow', as it were – aims to capture latent visibility properties of floorplans that emphasise how care staff can remain visually connected both to patients and to one another.

In her research, which was inspired by her former career as a nurse practitioner, Ossmann has identified correlations between her measure, 'Isovist Connectivity', and significant reductions in intensive care unit (ICU) mortality. She argues that 'finer-grained' measures should replace gross typological categories in researching and assessing the relative safety of acute-care nursing unit layout proposals.

George Tingwald, in his response essay, describes his personal experience supporting a loved one during an ICU stay, an experience that unfolded against his background as a medical doctor and hospital architect. He notes that even as innovative approaches to ICU design are advocated (e.g., in-room charting and same-handed rooms), effective ICU care will always support both nurse surveillance and teamwork, while also affirming the humanity of patients through privacy, quiet and the ability to keep loved ones close.

The patient and the reciprocal view

Michelle Ossmann

In the 30-plus years since researchers began to interrogate how organisational structure and process interacts with clinical treatments and interventions to influence patient outcomes, the built environment (a component of structure)[1] remains understudied and untapped. Contemporary architecture and interiors health research is much like nursing research in the late 1990s, where 'the components and outcomes of nursing care are buried in existing health services research as nonspecific features of organizational structure, or they may be the sole focus of nursing administration research'.[2] At that time, the state of the scholarship and implementation was such that the American Academy of Nursing convened an invitational conference to identify and clarify outcomes that were known or had the potential to be sensitive to organisational structure and recommend areas for development and research. As part of the discussion between health service researchers, nursing investigators, healthcare purchasers and policy makers, Mitchell and Shortell[3] asked a set of well-considered questions of the extant literature and, indeed, of all health researchers:

1. Why would one think that organisational features could affect mortality and other adverse events?
2. Is there any evidence to support current conceptual models?
3. To what extent are differences in mortality, morbidity and other adverse events among institutions reflective of differences in organisational structures and processes?

4. Do these differences disappear when clinical factors are accounted for adequately?
5. Is mortality an adequate proxy for other adverse events?

These queries could not be more appropriate for architects, interior designers, environmental psychologists and evidence-based design practitioners, as we similarly suffer from a state of absolute belief and a dearth of evidentiary outcomes. One need only review major medical and nursing journals and conference proceedings to see that the health design community is also in an echo-chamber; our scholarship rarely overlaps. All is not lost, however; before us is the opportunity to identify and clarify known relationships between built environment variables – components of structure and associated processes and outcomes – and moreover, determine which outcomes matter.[4] Mortality and adverse events are certainly the penultimate outcomes, commensurate with *prima non nocere*, 'first, do no harm'; arguably the most critical relationships to establish an 'understanding of' are those that are deleterious. But we have moved beyond harm in health-service research to acknowledge a broader accounting of healthcare quality. Such a shift is seen in measures such as patients' reported quality of life and financial impact.

Regardless of the chosen outcomes, the ability to measure the built environment component in question remains a fundamental issue (see Figure 2.1). We cannot overstate this importance, as the ability to describe, define and rigorously measure is that which allows for scientific advancement. Indeed, a lack of measurement may explain the siloed state of our field.[5] In this spirit, let us add to Mitchell and Shortell: (6) How does one measure the built environment?

While we might explore these six questions with any number of built-environment influences and outcomes,[6] this chapter will focus on a particular aspect of ICU patient safety:[7] clinical surveillance and the underpinning of surveillance that is environmentally afforded: visibility.

As a nurse in emergency departments and then a nurse practitioner in neurocritical care, I have personally prevented unplanned extubations and patients falling out of bed based on visual happenstance. I have halted unwitting medical errors by staff members while on the way to another task. I have carefully positioned myself both within eyesight and earshot of a tenuous patient and the corridor beyond to make sure that I caught the cardiologist. I have written discharge orders requiring 'a room in front of the nurse station' before permitting my patient to leave the ICU. But this goes beyond my personal experience – there is a lore among clinicians about patient rooms. Every nurse and doctor knows that some

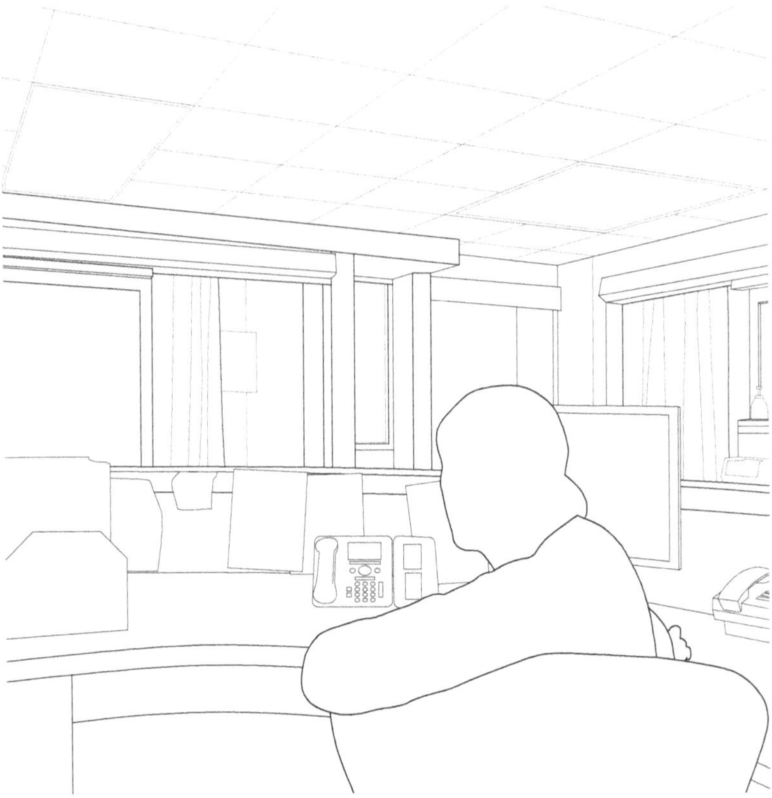

2.1 The patient-nurse visual link is critical for safety, but it has been difficult to fully understand how it works. Drawn by Victor Carrillo and Daniel Rios, 2021.

rooms are better than others; there are rooms that they would never wish to occupy. ICU staff have been known to move patients within the ICU to bring them closer to work areas when possible. Even patients who are unfortunate enough to become familiar with the inner workings of inpatient care know that space matters (see Figures 2.2a and 2.2b).[8] One emergency physician[9] shared his patient's reticence to be placed in the back hall of the emergency department, exclaiming, 'Doc, people die back there!' Thus far, the nursing and medical communities lacked the evidence to begin to confirm or refute what one could call magical thinking. Again, only rigorous measurement would allow such a conversation to commence.

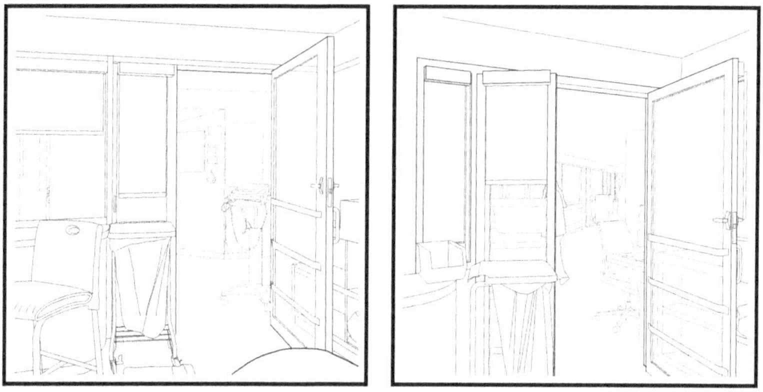

2.2a and 2.2b From the patient head of bed, different conditions for patient visibility. Drawn by Victor Carrillo and Daniel Rios, 2021.

Conceptualising surveillance

Contemporary acute or ICU patient care hinges on a central safety practice – clinical surveillance.[10] Surveillance is conceptualised as both a behavioural and cognitive process that involves the collection of primary and secondary sources of data.[11] Patient inspection – at the bedside or from a team station – palpation, auscultation and conversation are forms of primary patient data. Secondary data comes from digital or technical equipment and devices, family members and other clinical colleagues. The cognitive component includes active observing and monitoring, interpreting, analysing and synthesising these data types to identify potential threats to patient safety – prevention and response is the goal. As opposed to a single assessment[12] that is time-limited and episodic,[13] surveillance is continuous and performed with attention and vigilance.[14]

The round-the-clock nature of patient care means that surveillance takes place across and between clinical roles in the form of formal and informal handoffs.[15] The latter is of interest here. Nurses will ask of each other, 'Can you keep an eye on my patients while I —?' Routine care is not in the request; rather, in the swooping from task to task, the supporting nurse looks for the awry, moving on when none is found. Although surveillance is an 'assigned nursing responsibility', the behavioural and cognitive dimensions of surveillance are often operationalised within and across discipline in the form of general awareness, especially regarding sentinel[16] (i.e., patient safety) events.[17] In addition to providing more 'eyes on the patient', general awareness is the precursor to the situation monitoring, mutual support, communication and leadership that are critical to team performance.[18]

While surveillance is notionally a codified intervention, the mental and behavioural work is, in practice and perhaps at its best, an intuitive habit. In an acquired behaviour pattern, the expert clinician[19] uses their education, experience and intuition[20] to discriminate between signal and noise and take appropriate collaborative action, works to prevent untoward outcomes. Notably, Cynthia Dougherty recognises a sensorial component to surveillance, commenting that 'Perception and the ability to relate sensory stimuli to a knowledge base or to a previous experience are two essential elements of surveillance'.[21] Relating sensorially derived stimuli to developing or existing knowledge is key to developing pattern recognition, a critical element of expert nursing[22] and medical practice. But the habit – and indeed, surveillance becomes a habit – moves beyond answering immediate questions. Surveillance is a theory generating practice.[23] Through surveillance, clinicians develop a sense of the body's tendencies, a person's preferences and signs of concern and improvement. This intuition is fostered at the level of the individual and conducted in service of the population of patients one serves. Staff respond reflexively to the pattern of a patient edging towards the side of the bed, even when in passing to an unrelated task.

In recent years, nursing theorists have sought to conceptualise the individual and organisational features[24] or more specifically, antecedents[25] that must be present for proper surveillance. To differentiate between the individual and that which is external to the individual, we might consider these antecedents as intrinsic or extrinsic. Intrinsic antecedents (relating to individual characteristics of the nurse) include expertise (the confluence of education, experience and knowledge), intuition and early recognition skills. Extrinsic antecedents (relating to characteristics of the organisation or work environment) include staffing adequacy, skill mix, work or patient load and practice environment. Numerous studies have related both intrinsic and extrinsic surveillance antecedents to patient outcomes.[26] For example, in a landmark study of 10,184 nurses and 232,342 surgical patients in Pennsylvania, care environments,[27] nurse staffing and nurse education were significantly associated with failure to rescue and 30-day mortality.[28] Most recently, Lake and colleagues[29] completed an international meta-analysis of all studies completed between 2002 and 2018 investigating the influence of the nurse practice environment and reported a significant association on a broad range of outcomes, including nurse outcomes, safety and quality ratings, patient outcomes and patient satisfaction.

No doubt my fellow design colleagues read the term 'nurse practice environment' and presume a built environment reference. In nursing literature, however, practice environment typically refers to the organisational characteristics of a work setting such as leadership support, resources and nurse-physician relationships that help or hinder professional nursing practice. The only spatially descriptive antecedent is 'proximity to patients'[30] in Kelly and Vincent's nursing surveillance concept analysis, but the authors do not provide additional detail or propose measurement. Neither patient room location on the floorplan nor physical proximity to those with adjacent skill sets or supporting infrastructure are typically part of tools or consensus statements such as the *ANAs Principles for Nurse Staffing*.[31] Indeed, while a robust body of evidence details the positive relationship between nurse staffing and patient outcomes,[32] 'layout' is occasionally mentioned but not operationalised.[33] Differences in physical characteristics between units are often combined with other unit specific variables such as 'care delivery models' or ancillary staff availability as 'unit fixed effects',[34] or are subsumed by large, state-wide[35] or multi-state data sets.[36]

Although there is little to no mention of the built environment, layout (the organisation of rooms and connecting spaces) or visibility as an extrinsic surveillance antecedent in nursing literature,[37] interdisciplinary studies from human factors, systems engineering and architectural fields note a potentia impeding or beneficial antecedent. For example, nurses comment that 'Patients' rooms not close to each other'[38] and 'Layout not conducive to patient care'.[39] Evidence suggests a relationship between layout and process outcomes such as the length of time and frequency with which a nurse enters a patient room,[40] influencing patient observation[41] and staff communication.[42] For example, chest-pain patients located more than 25 feet from the physician workstation or who had a door on their rooms were significantly more likely to wait more than 10 minutes for their initial physician assessment.[43]

While initially puzzling, the lack of conceptual relationship between layout or visibility and surveillance in nursing literature may be because the ideal surveillance scenario is one in which the nurse is not required to leave the patient for any reason. Indeed, Dresser[44] illustrates this notion with contrasting case studies set in an ICU. As a 'model' example, the nurse is exceedingly well-qualified, anticipates all patient-care needs and remains with the patient continuously. By comparison, the 'contrary case' describes a less-experienced nurse whose support team is pulled away by other patient emergencies and for whom necessary supplies are not immediately available, requiring the attending nurse to leave the bedside.

In short, the contrary case describes the realities of acute patient care.[45] Henneman and colleagues' case study depicting surveillance activities for a sepsis patient similarly focuses all attention to nurse placement at the bedside,[46] as does Dougherty's[47] classic surveillance piece. It appears that the discourse on nurse surveillance has not only neglected the concept of physical environment but is also so schematic as to resemble fiction rather than likely working conditions. None of these case studies – ideal or otherwise – mentions the nurse having responsibility for another patient, supervising another nurse's patients while they are off the unit or engaging in self-care of any kind.

Albeit conceptually unacknowledged, early recommendations for ICU design by a collaboration between the Society for Critical Care Medicine and the American Association of Critical-Care Nurses tacitly recognised that the patient will not always have bedside surveillance and explicitly privilege visibility as an antecedent of the cognitive components of surveillance, stating:

> Patients must be situated so that direct or indirect (e.g., by video monitor) visualization by healthcare providers is possible at all times. This approach permits the monitoring of patient status under both routine and emergency circumstances. The preferred design is to allow a direct line of vision between the patient and the central nursing station. In ICUs with a modular design, patients should be visible from their respective nursing substations.[48]

An additional barrier to the exploration of a layout or visibility antecedent may be methodological. Even if intuitively relevant for surveillance and patient safety, how might clinical leadership rigorously measure layout or visibility? Catrambone[49] sought to quantify the various design characteristics deemed desirable by the Agency for Healthcare Research and Quality 2007 initiative, *Transforming Hospitals: Designing for Safety and Quality*. The authors measured 'visibility' of patients from nurse work areas by standing at each nurse charting area (i.e., station) and counting the number of beds where the upper third of the patient could be seen when the door or room blinds were open.[50] In 2010, Leaf and colleagues reported that severely ill patients[51] who were admitted to low-visibility rooms experienced significantly higher ICU mortality than those admitted to high-visibility rooms (66.7 per cent and 46.7 per cent respectively; $p = 0.042$). Although this finding was groundbreaking to those who study and design space, visibility was ascertained by looking for any part of the patient from the central nurse station. In both cases, the visibility measure was subjectively obtained, and we cannot know whether the observer leaned or strained to gain a more advantageous view or whether observations were truly taken from every available point in the nurse station. Nonetheless, Leaf and colleagues'[52] work influenced the 2012 SCCM Guidelines update,[53] as the authors comment: 'There is perhaps no better way of monitoring a patient than by direct visualization.' The update specifies that the face and body position should be easily seen from the corridor or team station and notes the benefit of visualisation from more than one team station.

We appear to have a mismatch between surveillance theory and practice, worsened by a lack of measurement capabilities. Nursing theorists and guidelines have detailed the thought processes, activities and antecedents for surveillance, but in keeping with most clinical literature, do not acknowledge the embodied nature of human perceptual-cognitive processes or the physical settings that frame human interaction. When clinicians are forced to consider architectural implications on surveillance practice, such affordances are desired but cannot be accurately described. And finally, the lack of fine-tuned measurement prevents the development of the knowledge base to affect theory in the first place. While one cannot always measure what matters, a refined measurement is required to advance scientific theory and enquiry and begin a rejoinder to the prescient question inspired by Mitchell and Shortell:[54] to what extent are differences in mortality, morbidity and other adverse events among institutions reflective of differences in the built environment?

Measuring what matters

Examples in literature suggest that built environment surveillance antecedents matter to patient outcomes, but clinical scholars lack spatial theory and tools to robustly evaluate this relationship. It is perhaps at this juncture in the history of surveillance antecedents that we introduce a parallel path of architectural scholarship that provides for fine-grained spatial analyses: environmental perception and spatial networks. For if visually related antecedents to surveillance are to be examined for their relationship to patient outcomes, rigorous measurement must be possible.

Environmental perception

Built upon the work of Tandy[55] and grounded in visual perception theory[56], Benedikt[57] sought to measure spatial experience and perception. Benedikt defined environmental perception as specific to the path along

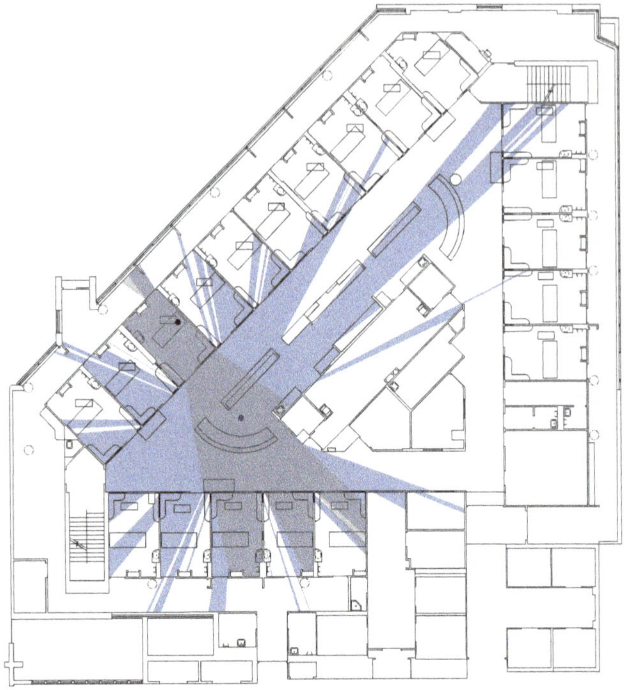

2.3 Isovist polygons (360°) as described by Benedikt (1979); generated from a patient bed (black point, grey field) and a nurse station (blue point and field). Drawn by Victor Carrillo and Daniel Rios, 2021.

which an individual observes information about the surrounding environment, measured from points along the given path. Stated geometrically, the area (and perimeter) visible around a point constitutes a closed polygon in interior settings;[58] this polygon is termed an 'isovist' (see Figure 2.3). This polygon or isovist provides information for the individual at each occupied vantage point, v_i, and the observed information shifts with movement to new points.

Although Benedikt's primary interest was the observer or vantage point perspective, v_i, an isovist informational field is also reciprocal to v_i – from any point within the polygon visible to v_i, v_i is also visible. Simply put, 'if I can see you, you can see me'. The reciprocal nature of isovists allows a change of perspective; instead of being concerned with the view from 'v_i', we may focus on all points within the polygon from which visual connection may be maintained with 'v_i' – that is, the neighbourhood. The notion of reciprocal informational fields is a critical methodological step for measuring the antecedents of clinical surveillance. The patient is the vantage point, v_i, and the polygon generated from the patient contains all

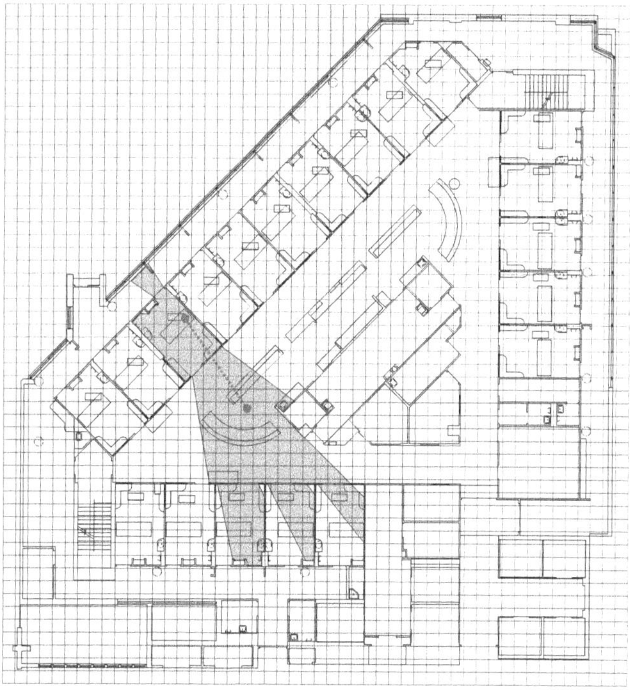

2.4 Visual connectivity graph example. Drawn by Victor Carrillo and Daniel Rios, 2021.

the places in the ICU where a clinician might maintain direct observation of that patient. In addition, the size and shape of an isovist approximates the amount of information available to and about the individual at v_i. A narrow, short isovist could yield very little information, while a long, wide isovist could reveal significantly more.

Spatial networks

Grounded in Hillier and Hanson's[59] graph-based theories on the social implications of inhabited, arranged spaces and Benedikt's description of an isovist, Turner and colleagues conceptualised the visibility graph of an environment: 'the graph of mutually visible locations in a spatial layout.'[60] To conduct a visibility graph analysis (VGA),[61] a graph is first constructed based on visibility polygons of all available visible locations from each point of an underlying grid or from pre-established points of special interest. Each visible location is a vertex or vantage point (v_i) and connections are made between pairs of vertices if they are mutually visible,[62] (see Figure 2.4).

Once every possible connection is made for every vertex or location, the visibility graph of the system is complete. Note, that by this definition, the visibility graph is fundamentally dependent on Benedikt's isovist. This set of immediate connections from each vertex point is a local measure, practically equivalent to the isovist, and called visual connectivity.[63]

While these advancements in spatial analyses may appear overly academic, they are critical because they allow the designer to mathematically describe the building's potential. How often have we encountered flowery language proclaiming the liveliness of a design? Rather, these measures and metrics allow both the future occupant and architect or designer to compare layout iterations with programmatic wishes and, perhaps most importantly, cross-compare built and occupied spaces to improve the social performance of future designs. Let us now explore the meaning of spatial measures and metrics.

Relating spatial metrics with behaviour and outcomes

Across an array of built environment settings – museums, offices, hospitals and other institutional environments – connectivity (and other spatial metrics) is associated with visual awareness, the presence of people, unplanned encounters and movement across space.[64] But the generic[65] spatial metrics that were so useful in predicting museum and office behaviour did not appear to replicate in ICU settings. In a first attempt to solve this puzzle, I studied the distribution patterns of clinical staff members in a neuroscience ICU together with colleagues.[66] We found no particular pattern of distribution demonstrating a preference for certain spaces that would favour clinician-specific behaviours, surveillance-related or otherwise.

After reflecting on these rather puzzling results, I hypothesised that generic measures failed because they did not capture ICU nurses' organising focus: the patient head of bed. Subsequently Lu and colleagues[67] used the same data set and built on this notion of surveillance and awareness with a new metric: targeted visibility. The running hypothesis was that because nurses and doctors are interested in a specific target – the patient head of bed – during movement through space, the ability to see more heads of bed at one time is preferable. Targeted visibility[68] values (TVi) ranged from 0–9, according to the number of heads of bed it was possible to view at one time. In general, physicians appeared to prefer locations with higher connectivity scores (higher general awareness potential, rather than targeted to patients), appropriate to a broader supervisory and care role. Nurses displayed conflicting behaviour, preferring the concurrent affordance of high numbers of visible heads of bed (high targeted visibility) and general awareness (high connectivity) while interacting and showing no spatially attributable preference when not interacting.

While confounding to the 2009 research team, it is not entirely unexpected that Lu and colleagues were unable to account for the movement of non-interacting nurses. Nursing work is not strictly defined by worker-worker interaction, however critical. Instead, nurse-patient primacy in ICUs is organisationally reinforced with specific assignments, usually in ratios of 1:2 and dominated by surveillance as a core nursing intervention. As has already been established, neither patient room location on the floorplan nor physical proximity to those with adjacent skill sets or supporting infrastructure are part of the concept of nursing surveillance. Targeted visibility was also not significantly related to mortality rates[69] in a replication study of Leaf and colleagues' 2010 Medical Intensive Care Unit (MICU) study. It appears that the targeted visibility score may have been inflated due to the layout shape – long and narrow – implying significant but unrealised, visibility gains. For example, the targeted visibility metric includes areas of the nurse station that are at 51 feet from the head of bed. This finding suggests a distance limitation for visualisation-dependent interventions, such as surveillance.

In our replication study, we tested field of view, defined as the maximum viewing angle from the patient head to the nurse station and measured in degrees, and this predicted 33.5 per cent of the variance in ICU mortality for very ill patients,[70] confirming the importance of head-of-bed visibility. The underlying premise is directionally correct, as nurses and indeed other clinical staff sit and linger at team stations for documentation and consultatory purposes. However, the field of view metric also unintentionally captured the space before and beyond the nurse station. Therefore, beyond some notion of head-of-bed importance, the field-of-view interpretation is confounded. We cannot know the influence of the corridor; fundamentally, the informational quality of the visual polygon that extends from the patient head of bed remains undescribed. Nevertheless, for those patients in this racetrack arrangement of rooms and nurse station, a wider visual angle conferred an advantage.

Conceptualising concurrent visibility

Thus far, we have discussed the dimensions and antecedents of clinical surveillance and the relationship to clinical outcomes. We then reviewed the burgeoning evidence relating elements of layout and visibility (however crudely measured) to clinically relevant outcomes, noting the need for honed spatial metrics. After examining the initial set of more finely tuned metrics seeking to capture the effect of layout and visibility on behaviour and then clinical outcomes, we propose a new measure, concurrent visibility, and its associated metric, *Isovist Connectivity*.[71] Let us review the assumptions and rationale behind measure and metric, which are both logically and intuitively born.

1. ICU layouts organise patient visibility and staff co-visibility, but the visibility distribution is latent and, as it cannot be easily perceived or understood, is missing from conceptual models.
2. The distribution of patient visibility underpins surveillance (and includes cognitive and behavioural components, visible means and instruments).
3. The distribution of staff co-visibility underpins team performance (situation monitoring, mutual support, leadership and communication).[72]
4. Patient visibility and staff co-visibility are required concurrently for patient safety – concurrent visibility – because visibility affects surveillance and team performance.
5. Traditional syntactic structure (e.g., isovists, visual connectivity, mean depth) does not explain or capture concurrent visibility.

Therefore, we develop a measure of 'concurrent visibility' and a corresponding metric, isovist connectivity, and test isovist connectivity against a set of data to explore its relevance.

Measuring concurrent visibility

Two primary organisational considerations drive the desired experience in space for hospital settings: patient surveillance and organisational awareness.[73] Traditional syntactic methods capture each individually, for example patient visibility in the isovist or field of view and staff co-visibility in connectivity. Each are insufficient in isolation, however, to capture the dual requirements of clinical care. The isovist speaks to patient visibility by identifying all the places a clinician may locate and maintain direct visualisation of the patient but does not capture visual access to co-workers or patterns of movement because the isovist does not differentiate spatial quality, for example, a space in front of the nurse station versus a space behind a door. Connectivity reflects the degree to

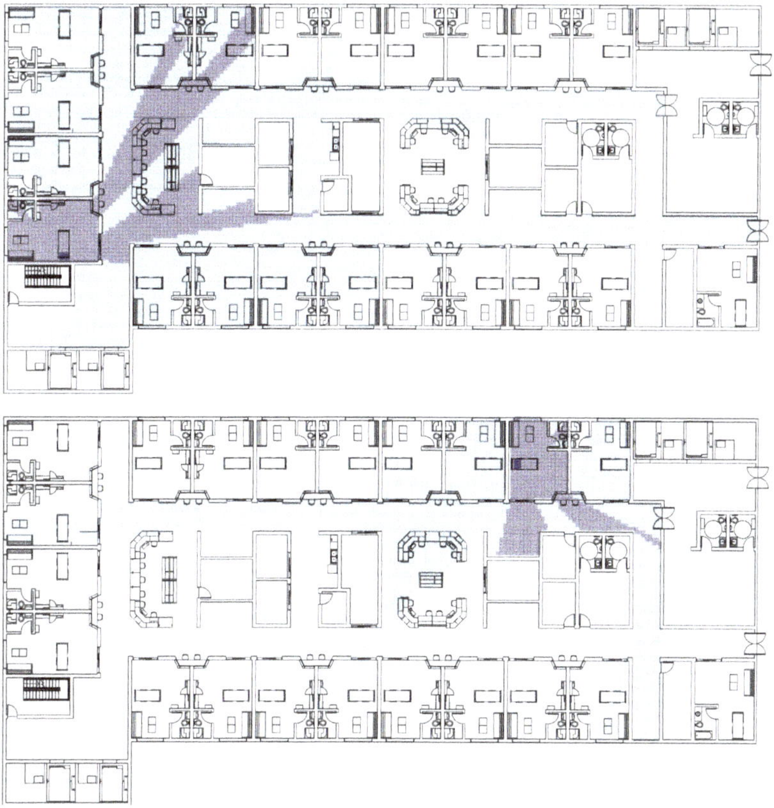

2.5a and 2.5b Concept diagram of the principle of isovist connectivity. The purple area is visible from the patient head of bed, while the blue is the area that can see some part of the purple. The larger the overall area, the better the capacity of the nurse to keep the patient in view while remaining visually connected to the rest of the unit. Diagram by Victor Carrillo and Daniel Rios, 2021.

which co-workers are visually available to each other and suggests patterns of local movement but does not account for a patient focus – all points are wholly considered equally.

Isovist connectivity[74] is defined for a single vantage point (v_i) although a set of directly adjacent vantage points may be chosen to enlarge the vantage point, such as the head of bed. Notionally, the isovist connectivity of a given vantage point, v_i, is the area of the visual polygon that is visible from anywhere within the isovist of v_i. For the purposes of nursing surveillance, there is an area of the patient care floor within which the nurse may move and yet maintain line of sight with the patient head of bed. Isovist connectivity captures all the additional places the nurse *may also see* while remaining in that patient-focused visual field. In other words, isovist connectivity reflects the potential for simultaneous, concurrent visibility to a patient of interest and the broader patient care floor (see Figures 2.5a and 2.5b). This means, effectively, that the isovist connectivity of a point is the average connectivity of all the points in the isovist of the point.

Testing isovist connectivity

In developing a test for isovist connectivity, it is useful to return once again to the extent to which the built environment reflects differences in mortality, morbidity and other adverse events among institutions. Do these differences disappear when clinical factors are accounted for adequately? The most significant impediment to health environment research is the frequent absence of a single set of variables: patient characteristics and acuity by room, whether as a predictor or outcome. Patient characteristics such as age and sex carry their own predictive value. In addition to predictive value, patient acuity draws resources and attention, and in terms of spatial affordances, may supersede programme and probabilistic movement. For example, unless acuity is accounted for in the statistical model, we cannot determine whether any differences in patient outcomes (in this case mortality) are due simply to the likelihood of survivability by diagnosis. But how to account for acuity in a medical-surgical ICU, which by design admits myriad patient types with any number of primary diagnoses?[75] The task was to find a sufficiently large and similar patient population where we could reliably and meaningfully account for severity of illness. Such was the rationale for selecting patients with a diagnosis of sepsis.[76] Not only do accepted acuity scales exist to quantify the severity of illness, but the medical and economic burdens associated with sepsis are enormous.[77]

A similar issue exists with the practice setting, as differences in intrinsic staff characteristics, staffing ratios, physician and ancillary coverage, care protocols and other practice work environment differences could create variation in outcomes. The single-centre cohort at Emory University Health System alleviated much of this variability, providing uniform medical and nursing staffing and credentialling requirements, advance practice provider coverage, rounding frequency, admission patterns and shift patterns.

The considerations for selecting the physical settings – or, more tactically speaking, a set of study floorplans – took the opposite

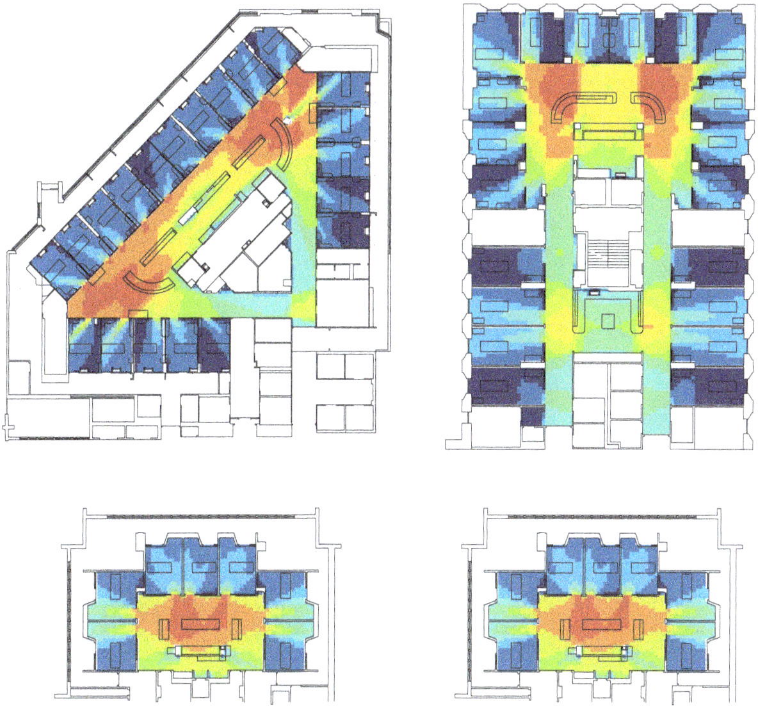

2.6 Visual connectivity graphs for four Emory intensive care units (ICUs): Unit A (top left) B (top right) and C and D (bottom row). Image by Michelle Ossmann, 2015.

approach.[78] Rather than hoping for typologically similar ICUs, we were fortunate that Emory University Health System[79] had within its portfolio three differentiated types of medical-surgical ICU: triangular (ICU A), U-shape (ICUs B and C) and double-corridor (ICU D).[80] Visual connectivity analyses of these units is shown in Figure 2.6.

This divergent set allows us to test the effect of isovist connectivity across layout type. The question of ideal inpatient layout type is frequently raised in architectural design and research – what is the ideal patient care unit configuration? In the United States, ICU design excellence has been awarded since 1993 by a joint effort of the Society of Critical Care Medicine, the American Academy of Critical Care Nurses and the American Institute of Architects. But since at least 2003, the last year for which a systematic assessment of the winning designs exists (as far as we are aware), no one configuration is demonstrably superior. Rashid[81] found seven different nurse station configurations among four differing unit layout typologies; the most common (12 of 19) was 'racetrack'. In addition, there was variation in the number of patient rooms per unit, support service area locations and unit entrances. By examining the patient-care unit according to the desired *syntactic* experience in space[82] – that is, by the way the building empirically supports key clinical practices – we may begin to compare designs by experience rather than by typology.

With these criteria in mind, we explored the relationship between concurrent visibility and mortality. All adults with a sepsis discharge diagnosis who were admitted to Emory University Health System's ICUs A, B, C and D between 1 September 2011 and 30 June 2014[83] were eligible for study enrolment.[84] We calculated the isovist connectivity score for each patient room head of bed and used a hierarchical clustering method[85] to create groups of concurrent visibility – low, medium and high[86] (see Figure 2.7). For the binary outcome variable 'ICU mortality', we performed a multivariate logistic regression analysis to assess the association between isovist connectivity group (low, medium and high) and ICU mortality, adjusting for age, gender, ventilation days and severity

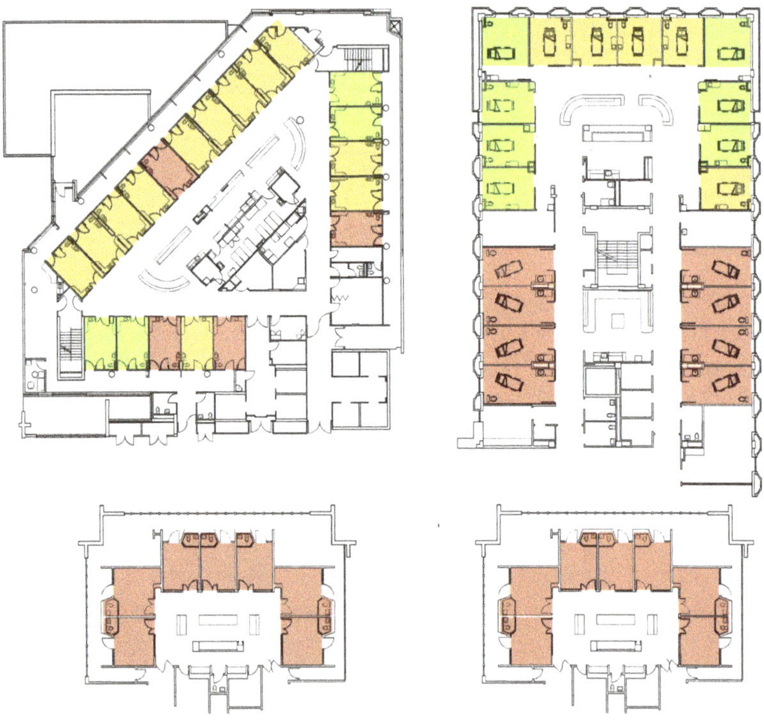

2.7 High (green), medium (gold) and low (red) isovist connectivity values for patient rooms in four ICUs. Image by Victor Carrillo and Daniel Rios, 2021.

of illness,[87] with a p value of less than 0.05 considered statistically significant. The adjusted odds ratio with 95 per cent CI (confidence interval) is reported. This study was approved by the Emory Institutional Review Board.

In this study, patients exposed to a high isovist connectivity score room experienced a 42 per cent (95 per cent CI, 0.33–0.99) lower odds of death compared to patients exposed to a low isovist connectivity score room, $p = 0.048$. Patients in medium visibility rooms trended similarly but did not achieve statistical significance. In short, patients with a diagnosis of sepsis admitted to rooms with a high isovist connectivity score were less likely to die.[88]

Discussion: towards an integration of clinical and architectural expertise

Surveillance is a core function for nursing and other clinical staff. But as the healthcare industrial complex evolved, first from Hill-Burton supplying the design and construction of hospitals across the United States, and then from large to smaller patient wards and then double to single occupancy patient rooms, the number of patients that a single nurse could observe at one time decreased ten-fold. The resultant visual and auditory privacy and environmental control of infectious agents, to say nothing of the financial improvements associated with higher occupancy rates of single rooms are significant. But these changes – walls, doors, occupancy patterns – altered the distribution of patient visibility.

Team or nurse station design adjusted accordingly. While team stations tucked in lengths of corridor functioned to serve patient bays with multiple patients and paper-based documentation, clinicians and architects recognised a change was needed to gather people, paperwork and computers. But the patient did not centralise with the work. Decentralised stations are at once lauded and maligned, for while the nurse is anchored to the bedside, they are isolated from the learning community of practice. Clinicians and architects must surely wonder, is it always 'or', is it never 'and'? Perhaps the first step is moving to *sensorial* design, rather than by programme. Consider a design framework that prioritises the underpinnings of nearly all clinical endeavours – to see, to hear, to smell, to touch. And as with the isovist, these sensorial traits are not clinician-only; patients also see and hear others, smell and touch.[89] What novel solution might such an approach produce?

The concept of concurrent visibility was developed as the measure of 'isovist connectivity' based on a deep understanding of both clinician work and spatial morphology. First, the isovist geometry accounts for the visual antecedents of patient surveillance. Second, the connectivity measure captures the antecedents of receiving and providing inter-professional and intra-professional support and general awareness of others. However, this is only the first examination of the relationship between concurrent visibility and its metric, isovist connectivity. Further questions arise – for example, on external validity. Do similar results occur with sepsis patients in other health systems, with different patient populations or with floorplans that vary by size and typology?

We do have some indication of isovist connectivity's construct validity; fundamentally isovist connectivity is a measure of the informational potential of the isovist around v_i. Replicating my method, a subsequent study by Joshi used isovist connectivity[90] to measure the degree of emergency physician (v_i) visual exposure to the rest of the department while seated in three different workstation enclosure types as a predictor of interruptions during patient handoffs. Among other results, the number of interruptions per hour were significantly higher in locations with high isovist connectivity scores compared to locations with medium ($p = 0.0009$) and low scores ($p = 0.0015$). This finding was consistent with emergency physicians' perception of interruption; more physicians in high isovist connectivity workstations perceived they were interrupted than those in low isovist connectivity workstations. Perceived privacy followed similar patterns, as 88 per cent of the incoming and outgoing physicians in the low isovist connectivity locations agreed that they had privacy to document and discuss, whereas only 43 per cent in medium and 8 per cent in high isovist connectivity locations felt the same.

Interesting statistical inferences aside, Joshi's work was targeted at a specific, long-standing architectural problem: our penchant for conflating type and form. When one is simply seeking to describe, or perhaps use as a general precedent, workstations classified as open, semi-open and closed may suffice. Once one wishes to generate a hypothesis and expect an outcome, overlapping and flexible categories reduce the strength of association. Moreover, the discursive gets firmly in the way; is the workstation semi-open or semi-closed? If architecture and design wish to cross into clinical literature, taught in nursing and medical schools as critical practice factors affecting the outcomes of their patients, then these finer-grained metrics must be used to articulate the differences between designs. Isovist connectivity is but one of several movements in this direction, and while a significant step towards answering Mitchell and Shortell's question has been achieved, much opportunity lies ahead.

Response Essay: The evolution of surveillance in ICU design

George Tingwald

The invention of the ICU had as its two most fundamental tenets the cohorting of critically ill patients and specially trained staff and clinical surveillance achieved by maximal visibility of the patient. Its impact on morbidity and mortality was immediate and profound. And while the principles of cohorting and surveillance have not changed, the relationship of surveillance to visibility has changed fundamentally due to advances in organisational structure, profound shifts in patient and family advocacy, and the ever-increasing pace of technological advancement. I have had the great privilege over the past year of seeing the opening of the new ICUs at Stanford Hospital that I planned and designed over a 10-year period together with the unexpected need to spend a month there taking care of my critically ill wife. These professional and personal events reached their extrema during a pandemic that tested all the innovations built into the new design and will be the catalyst for the most fundamental changes in healthcare since, possibly, the invention of the ICU.

Our patient journey started at the ICU of the hospital closest to our home, a facility that was planned more than 40 years ago and was truly state of the art at that time. The unit was primarily open bays with direct visibility to a central nursing station. While there was visible privacy provided by curtains, there was no auditory privacy at all. My wife, an emergency medicine physician, was certainly more familiar and comfortable with this setting than the average patient. Due to COVID-19, no visitors were allowed. Alone in a curtained space, she could not orientate herself to person, place or time of day. Her status deteriorated quickly, she was diagnosed with septic shock and, most alarming to me, she developed profound ICU psychosis. After five days, she was transferred to Stanford, a move we both agree saved her life. While the expertise of the medical staff and the outstanding nursing care were the most important elements of her successful recovery, the physical environment of care played a profound role. Stanford Hospital was designed with a commitment to patients and families first, and while the hospital increased restrictions, they never eliminated family visitation during the pandemic. I am confident that this policy significantly decreased my wife's morbidity and shortened her length of stay in the ICU and hospitalisation overall. I worked with the staff to reorientate my wife to time and place during the 12 hours I was allowed to be there each day, and through technology her sister, thousands of miles away, took the night shift. At Stanford, the family is now part of the surveillance proposition in the ICU, not just the nursing and medical staff. Recognising the surveillance potential of family has changed the physical design of the unit in many ways.

One of the first steps in designing the new ICUs was a series of visits to recently completed units at comparable institutions. We were fortunate to have two units of similar size and acuity, only miles apart in Los Angeles, and they could not have been more different. Cedars Sinai's new Critical Care Tower had patient rooms that looked essentially like a modified standard acute care room, with the ability to be used for non-critical care use if the census allowed. UCLA Ronald Reagan Medical Center had patient rooms that looked more like operating rooms, with glass everywhere providing maximum visibility, and overhead equipment booms. We made two initial visits, the first with board members and donors, many of whom had had personal or family experiences in the ICU, including deaths. They uniformly preferred the Cedars Sinai model, with significant negative reactions to the other model due to acoustics, lack of patient privacy and limited space and accommodations for family rooming-in. In short, they found the environment terrifying. The second visit included physician and nursing leadership, who uniformly preferred the UCLA Reagan model. The design team clearly had a predicament on their hands, and the challenge was clear: how to create an environment that met the clinical requirements identified by the staff, but in a way that put the patient and families first.

The first major decision was to base the overall layout of the ICUs and the acute care units on the same basic room module and configuration.

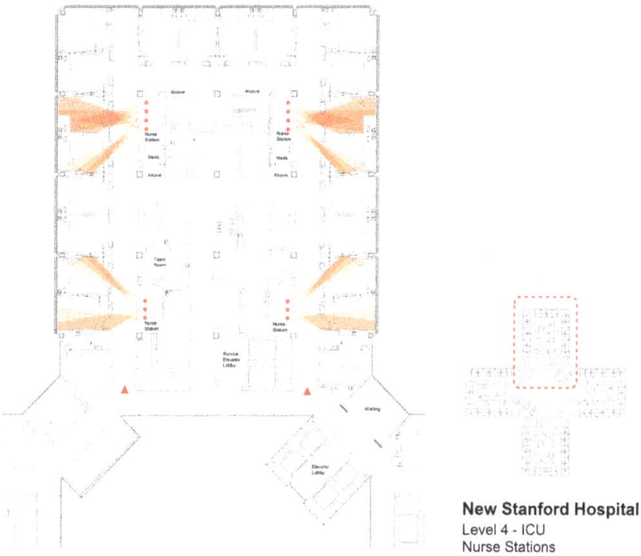

2.8 Nurse sub-station and visibility to patient rooms. Courtesy of Stanford Health Care.

This allowed for the creation of universal rooms (within code restrictions), meaning the two types of unit could adapt to either increasing or decreasing patient acuity with the minimum amount of reconfiguration. This was obtainable due to new technologies in construction that meet fire-rating requirements for glass doors and walls in the corridors of the ICUs. Now, when you enter the ICU, it has the look, sound and feel of any other unit in the hospital.

Both unit types have taken the traditional central nursing station and divided it into four sub-stations at the four corners of the unit (see Figure 2.8). While this is often called 'decentralised nursing', it is important to understand that it is a modification, not an elimination, of the traditional team-based model. Some nursing theorists have taken the advent of bedside electronic charting as the catalyst for an ideal surveillance scenario, where the nurse remains with the patient continuously, eliminating the need for centralised stations altogether. This concept is a theoretical fantasy, even in the most highly staffed units, such as Stanford. One of the things that I learned through direct observation is that one-to-one nursing care, meaning one nurse assigned to only one patient, does not equate to continuous direct patient observation, despite hearing this from countless nurses in planning sessions over the years. Furthermore, as a family member, I was glad that the nursing staff were only in the room when necessary, rather than continuously. While the Stanford design has bedside charting, it has also increased the capacity of centralised charting, finally providing access for all members of the care team. This design provides direct surveillance of every patient room, capturing both patient and co-worker visibility (conforming with Ossmann's high isovist connectivity). It also minimises travel distances to both charting and supplies.

Along with both bedside and central charting, the ICUs have a third location for nurse work, directly outside each patient room (see Figure 2.9). These charting alcoves provide direct staff visibility into two adjacent patient rooms without creating any visibility between rooms. Certain room designs, responding to nursing requests, provided either windows or sliding glass doors between adjacent rooms to increase visibility and access between adjacent rooms: a fallback to the days of open bay ICUs. Over time these have proven to be poorly, if ever, utilised, as well as acting as significant obstacles to patient and family privacy. The alcove, however, responds to this very real challenge of supporting surveillance of high-acuity patients when continuous in-room observation is not practical. It also meets the code requirements for direct observation from a nursing

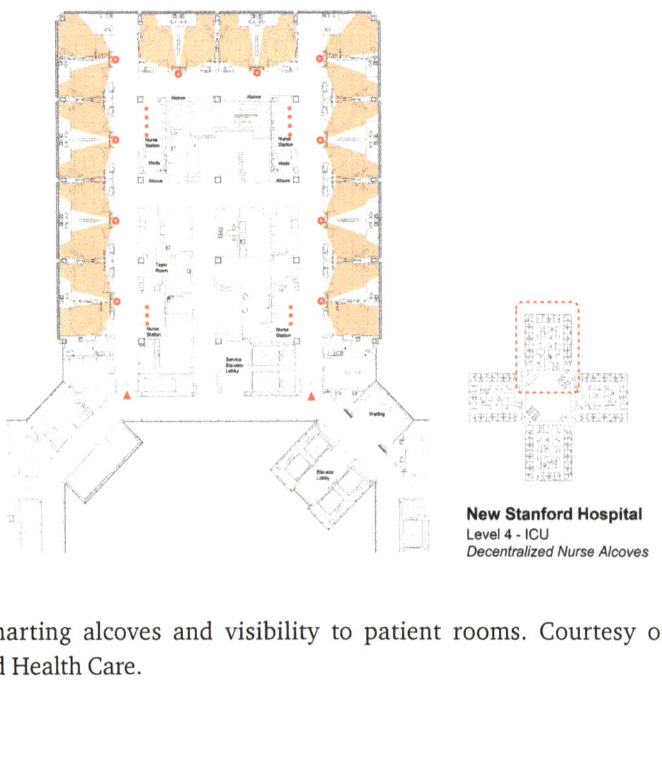

2.9 Charting alcoves and visibility to patient rooms. Courtesy of Stanford Health Care.

station but, as stated earlier, should not be a substitute for centralised charting.

To provide these charting alcoves, it is necessary to 'mirror' two adjacent rooms. During the time of the design, there was a very active movement towards designing 'single-handed' rooms, meaning that all rooms should be identical in all aspects. This theory was based on evidence from other fields that variations in design lead to safety risks. At Stanford, we built full scale mock-ups of both single-handed and mirrored rooms to test this theory. The actual area around each patient bed was designed identically, but the overall room envelope was either identical or mirrored. We found no significant difference when surveying our staff, so we were confident in our ability to provide increased surveillance without compromising safety. This is just one example of the value of building mock-ups during the design process.

Almost all designs have unintended consequences, meaning that they are used in ways not predicted during the design process (see Figure 2.10). The charting alcoves have proven to be invaluable during the current COVID-19 pandemic. Nurses have moved their primary site of activity from the patient room to minimise cross-contamination. The ability to provide surveillance of the patient and have proximal technological support without significant construction has proven to be of enormous benefit. The engagement of the family has also been profoundly compromised. The 'no visitors' policies have had an immeasurable impact. Here is where recent advances in technology and communications have played such a major role and will continue to redefine how surveillance is provided. The bond between patients and families, and between care providers and families must be met, and the amazing advances in telecommunications over the past year may prove to be among the greatest unintended beneficial consequences of this horrible disease.

When designing an ICU from the patient and family-first perspective, it is absolutely fundamental for them to have a say in the process, both through direct engagement as experts on equal footing with the nurses, physicians and other staff, and through the advocacy of the design team to come up with solutions that work for both sides. Fundamentally, patients and families do not want to be in ICUs, they are terrified and want as much normality, dignity and privacy as possible. The acuity of their illness should not be an excuse for ignoring their basic humanity. They do not want to see or hear what is going on outside their room. They want to know who is looking in or entering their room at all times. They want to see outside, know what time of day it is and be able to

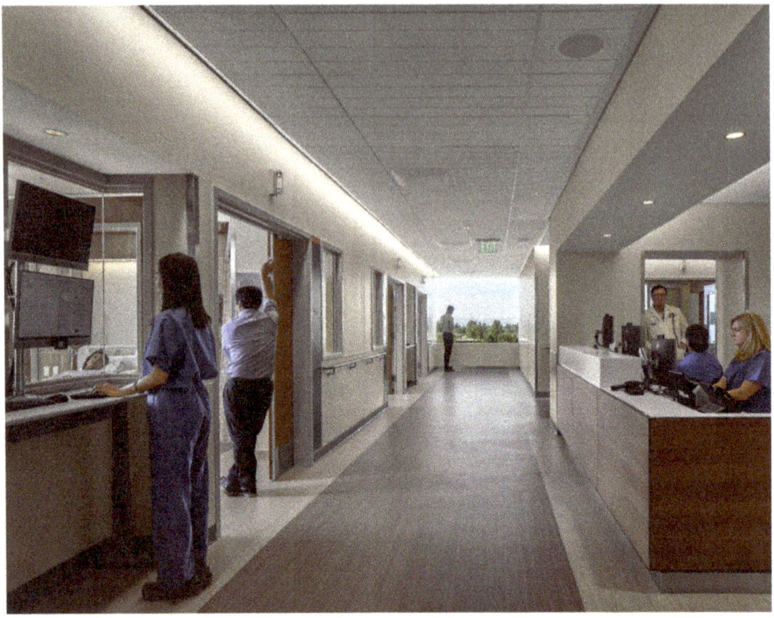

2.10 The charting alcoves were particularly useful during pandemic conditions. Courtesy of Stanford Health Care, image by Will Pryce.

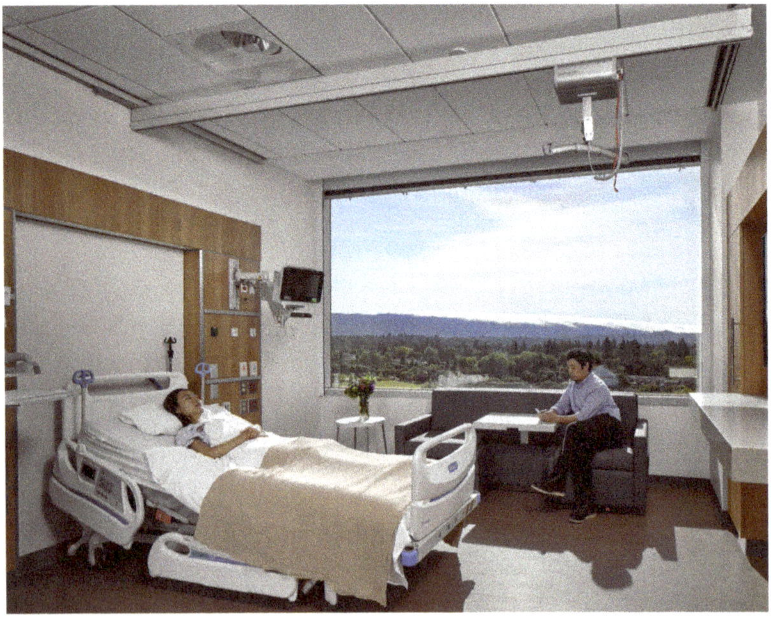

2.11 Patient rooms with outside views and places for extended community. Courtesy of Stanford Health Care, image by Will Pryce.

communicate with their extended community (see Figure 2.11). While surveillance is essential, it should not come at the expense of the patient and family experience. When I ask my wife what the most important differentiator of her Stanford experience was, she said it was that I was there, that she had an advocate.

Notes

1 Donabedian rather famously developed the framework by which care quality could be measured: 'structure' supports 'process', which leads to 'outcomes'. Holden built on this framework through human factors and a safety lens (assuming safety as the presumptive quality measure) but the underpinning is the same. In addition to physical infrastructure such as facilities, equipment and supplies, organisational and operational capabilities make up 'structure'. See Avedis Donabedian, 'The quality of care', *JAMA*, 260, no. 12 (1988), 1743–8; Richard J. Holden *et al.*, 'SEIPS 2.0: a human factors framework for studying and improving the work of healthcare professionals and patients', *Ergonomics*, 56, no. 11 (2013), 1669–86, https://doi.org/10.1080/00140139.2013.838643.
2 Pamela H. Mitchell, Jan Heinrich, Patricia Moritz and Ada Sue Hinshaw, 'Outcome measures and care delivery systems', *Medical Care*, 35, no. 11 (1997), 1–5, https://doi.org/10.1097/00005650-199711001-00001.
3 Pamela H. Mitchell and Steven M. Shortell, 'Adverse outcomes and variations in organization of care delivery', *Medical Care*, 35, no. 11 (1997), 19–32, https://doi.org/10.1097/00005650-199711001-00003.
4 Agency for Healthcare Research and Quality, Rockville, MD, 'Types of health care quality measures' (accessed 27 February 2021), https://www.ahrq.gov/talkingquality/measures/types.html; Center for Medicare and Medicaid Services, 'Meaningful measure hub', *Meaningful Measures Framework* (10 September 2019), https://www.cms.gov/Medicare/Quality-Initiatives-Patient-Assessment-Instruments/QualityInitiativesGenInfo/MMF/General-info-Sub-Page.
5 A lack of agreement is perhaps as damaging as the lack of measurement. As an example, for a number of years nursing researchers debated how nurse staffing might be defined and accounted for in outcomes models. Such variability makes drawing conclusions about the effect and importance of nurse staffing difficult.
6 Roger Ulrich, Craig Zimring, Xuemei Zhu, Jennifer DuBose, Hyun-Bo Seo, Young-Seon Choi, Xiaobo Quan and Anjali Joseph, 'A review of the research literature on evidence-based healthcare design', *HERD: Health Environments Research and Design Journal*, 1, no. 3 (2008), 61–125.
7 Institute of Medicine, Ann Page (ed.), 'Keeping patients safe: transforming the work environment of nurses' (Washington DC: National Academies Press, 2004), https://doi.org/10.17226/10851.
8 Stefnee J. Trzpuc and Caren S. Martin, 'Application of space syntax theory in the study of medical-surgical nursing units in urban hospitals', *HERD*, 4, no. 1 (2010), 34–55, https://doi.org/10.1177/193758671000400104.
9 Dr Bryan McNally, personal conversation, 2015.
10 Institute of Medicine, 2004.
11 Cynthia M. Dougherty, 'Surveillance', in Gloria M. Bulecheck and Joanne C. McCloskey (eds) *Nursing Interventions: Effective Nursing Treatments* (3rd edition), (St Louis MO: Elsevier, 1999), 524–32; Daniel Milhomme, Johanne Gagnon and Kathleen Lechasseur, 'The clinical surveillance process as carried out by expert nurses in a critical care context: a theoretical explanation', *Intensive and Critical Care Nursing*, 44 (2018), 24–30, https://doi.org/10.1016/j.iccn.2017.07.010.
12 One could conceptualise surveillance as a collection of individual assessments over time and across people.
13 Dougherty, 'Surveillance'.

14 Lesly Kelly and Deborah Vincent, 'The dimensions of nursing surveillance: a concept analysis', *Journal of Advanced Nursing*, 67, no. 3 (March 2011), 652–61, https://doi.org/10.1111/j.1365-2648.2010.05525.x.

15 Handoffs are an additional source of error. Dale M. Pfrimmer *et al.*, 'Surveillance', *Dimensions of Critical Care Nursing*, 36, no. 1 (2017), 45–52, doi:10.1097/dcc.0000000000000217.

16 A 'sentinel event' is a patient safety event that results in patient death, permanent or severe temporary harm; it is not primarily related to natural causes as relates to a patient's underlying illness or medical condition. The Joint Commission, 'Sentinel event', *Patient Safety Topics* (2021), https://www.jointcommission.org/resources/patient-safety-topics/sentinel-event/.

17 Milhomme, Gagnon and Lechasseur, 'The clinical surveillance process as carried out by expert nurses in a critical care context', 24–30.

18 Judith H. Heerwagen, Kevin Kampschroer, Kevin M. Powell and Vivian Loftness, 'Collaborative knowledge work environments', *Building Research and Information*, 32, no. 6 (2004), 510–28; Mahbub Rashid, 'Hospital design and face-to-face interaction among clinicians: a theoretical model', *HERD*, 2, no. 4 (2009), 62–84, https://doi.org/10.1177/193758670900200404; Carolyn M. Clancy and David N. Tornberg, 'TeamSTEPPS: assuring optimal teamwork in clinical settings', *American Journal of Medical Quality*, 22, no. 3 (2007), 214–17, https://doi.org/10.1177/1062860607300616.

19 Stuart E. Dreyfus, 'The five-stage model of adult skill acquisition', *Bulletin of Science, Technology and Society*, 24, no. 3 (2004), 177–81, https://doi.org/10.1177/0270467604264992; Patricia E. Benner, *From Novice to Expert: Excellence and Power in Clinical Nursing Practice* (Institute for Studies in Pragmaticism, 1984).

20 Kelly and Vincent, 'The dimensions of nursing surveillance'.

21 Dougherty, 'Surveillance'.

22 Benner, *From Novice to Expert*.

23 This generative practice occurs writ large and at the level of the individual patient. Together with empirical data, clinicians develop a theory of what went awry, how long it will take to improve and what will bring improvement.

24 Kutney-Lee and colleagues developed an organisational indicator – the Hospital Nurse Surveillance Capacity Profile (HNSCP) – to capture the dimensions affecting surveillance and, in turn, the relationship to patient outcomes. The HNSCP includes registered nurse characteristics (staffing, education, clinical expertise and years of experience) and the nurse practice environment. Ann Kutney-Lee, Eileen T. Lake and Linda H. Aiken, 'Development of the hospital nurse surveillance capacity profile', *Research in Nursing and Health*, 32, no. 2 (April 2009), 217–28, https://doi.org/10.1002/nur.20316.

25 Kelly and Vincent, 'The dimensions of nursing surveillance'.

26 Jack Needleman *et al.*, 'Association of Registered nurse and nursing support staffing with inpatient hospital mortality', *BMJ Quality and Safety*, 29, no. 1 (2020), 10, https://doi.org/10.1136/bmjqs-2018-009219; Linda H. Aiken, 'Hospital Nurse staffing and patient mortality, nurse burnout, and job dissatisfaction', *JAMA*, 288, no. 16 (23 October 2002), 1987, https://doi.org/10.1001/jama.288.16.1987; L. H. Aiken *et al.*, 'Effects of hospital care environment on patient mortality and nurse outcomes', *The Journal of Nursing Administration*, 38, no. 5 (2008), 223–9; Eileen T. Lake, Kathryn A. Riman and Douglas M. Sloane, 'Improved work environments and staffing lead to less missed nursing care: a panel study', *Journal of Nursing Management*, 28, no. 8 (2020), 2157–65, https://doi.org/10.1111/jonm.12970; Peter Griffiths *et al.*, 'Nurse staffing, nursing assistants and hospital mortality: retrospective longitudinal cohort study', *BMJ Quality and Safety*, 28, no. 8 (2019), 609, https://doi.org/10.1136/bmjqs-2018-008043.

27 Care environment is measured by the practice environment scale of the nursing work index (or 'PES-NWI'). E. T. Lake, 'Development of the practice environment scale of the nursing work index', *Res Nurs Health*, 25, no. 3 (2002), 176–88.

28 Aiken *et al.*, 'Effects of hospital care environment on patient mortality and nurse outcomes'.

29 Eileen T. Lake *et al.*, 'A meta-analysis of the associations between the nurse work environment in hospitals and 4 sets of outcomes', *Medical Care*, 57, no. 5 (2019), 353–61, https://doi.org/10.1097/mlr.0000000000001109.

30 Kelly and Vincent, 'The dimensions of nursing surveillance'.

31 American Nurses Association, 2012.

32 Paul G. Shekelle, 'Nurse-patient ratios as a patient safety strategy: a systematic review', *Annals of Internal Medicine*, 158, no. 5, Pt 2 (5 March 2013), 404–9, https://doi.org/10.7326/0003-4819-158-5-201303051-00007.

33 Avalere Health, LLC, 2015.

34 Jack Needleman *et al.*, 'Nurse staffing and inpatient hospital mortality', *N Engl J Med*, 364, no. 11 (17 March 2011), 1037–45, https://doi.org/10.1056/nejmsa1001025.

35 Aiken, 'Hospital nurse staffing and patient mortality, nurse burnout, and job dissatisfaction'.

36 Needleman *et al.*, 'Nurse staffing and inpatient hospital mortality'.

37 Clarke (2004) and Kalisch (2006) do refer to lack of proximity to patients in regard to missed care. See Beatrice J. Kalisch, 'Missed nursing care: a qualitative study', *Journal of Nursing Care and Quality*, 21, no. 4 (2006), 306–13; Sean P. Clarke, 'Failure to rescue: lessons from missed opportunity in care', *Nursing Inquiry*, 11, no. 2 (2004), 67–71.

38 Among a variety of performance obstacles, for example distractions, crowding and available equipment, nurses commented on layout. Ayse P. Gurses and Pascale Carayon, 'Performance obstacles of intensive care nurses', *Nursing Research*, 56, no. 3 (2007), 185, P. Carayon *et al.*, 'Work system design for patient safety: the SEIPS Model', *Quality and Safety in Health Care*, 15, no. suppl_1 (1 December 2006): 50–58, https://doi.org/10.1136/qshc.2005.015842.

39 Anita L. Tucker *et al.*, 'Front-line staff perspectives on opportunities for improving the safety and efficiency of hospital work systems', *Health Services Research*, 43, no. 5, pt 2 (2008), 1807–29, https://doi.org/10.1111/j.1475-6773.2008.00868.x.

40 Ann L. Hendrich, 'A 36-hospital time and motion study: how do medical-surgical nurses spend their time?', *The Permanente Journal*, 12, no. 3 (2008), 25–34; Yi Lu, 'Measuring the structure of visual fields in nursing units', *HERD* 3, no. 2 (2010), 48–59.

41 Ann L. Hendrich, Joy Fay and Amy K. Sorrells, 'Effects of acuity-adaptable rooms on flow of patients and delivery of care', *American Journal of Critical Care*, 13, no. 1 (2004), 35–45, https://doi.org/10.4037/ajcc2004.13.1.35.

42 Gurses and Carayon, 'Performance obstacles of intensive care nurses'; Rashid, 'Hospital design and face-to-face interaction among clinicians'.

43 Kendall K. Hall, Demetrios N. Kyriacou, Jonathan A. Handler and James G. Adams,, 'Impact of emergency department built environment on timeliness of physician assessment of patients with chest pain', *Environment and Behavior*, 40, no. 2 (2008), 233–48.

44 Susan Dresser, 'The role of nursing surveillance in keeping patients safe', *JONA*, 42, no. 7/8 (2012), 361–8, https://doi.org/10.1097/nna.0b013e3182619377.

45 This is not to imply that organiaations should not strive for prepared and well-supported nurses. Rather, that a preferred scenario might be one in which the system handles such stresses with minimal disruption and is resilient.

46 Elizabeth A. Henneman, Anna Gawlinski and Karen K. Giuliano, 'Surveillance: a strategy for improving patient safety in acute and critical care units', *Critical Care Nurse*, 32, no. 2 (31 March 2012), e9–18, https://doi.org/10.4037/ccn2012166.

47 Dougherty, 'Surveillance'.

48 S. Wedel *et al.*, 'Guidelines for intensive care unit design: guidelines/practice parameters committee of the American College of Critical Care Medicine, Society of Critical Care Medicine', *Critical Care Medicine*, 23, no. 3 (March 1995), 582–8.

49 Cathy Catrambone *et al.*, 'The design of adult acute care units in U.S. hospitals', *Journal of Nursing Scholarship*, 41, no. 1 (March 2009), 79–86, https://doi.org/10.1111/j.1547-5069.2009.01254.x.

50 The sample was 56 randomly selected metropolitan hospital ICUs and medical surgical units. Across eight different ICU design typologies, only 63.4 per cent (SD 31.2) of the top one-third of patient beds were seen when standing up at a nurse charting station, and no typology, layout, number of rooms or combination of support areas was superior in visibility. Catrambone, 'The design of adult acute care units in U.S. hospitals'.

51 Severely ill patients were categorised as having an Acute Physiology and Chronic Health Evaluation II (APACHE II) > 30. Low visibility rooms were those where no part of the patient could be seen from the central nurse station. David E. Leaf, Peter Homel and Phillip H. Factor, 'Relationship between ICU design and mortality', *Chest*, 137, no. 5 (May 2010), 1022–7, https://doi.org/10.1378/chest.09-1458.

52 Leaf, 'Relationship between ICU design and mortality'.

53 Dan R. Thompson *et al.*, 'Guidelines for intensive care unit design', *Critical Care Medicine*, 40, no. 5 (May 2012), 1586–600, https://doi.org/10.1097/ccm.0b013e3182413bb2.

54 Mitchell and Shortell, 'Adverse outcomes and variations in organization of care delivery'.
55 C. Tandy, 'The isovist method of landscape survey', in H. C. Murray (ed.), *Symposium: Methods of Landscape Analysis* (London: Landscape Research Group, 1967), 9–10.
56 James J. Gibson, *The Ecological Approach to Visual Perception* (London: Lawrence Erlbaum Associates, 1986).
57 M. L. Benedikt, 'To take hold of space: isovists and isovist fields', *Environment and Planning B: Planning and Design*, 6 (2 January 1979), 47–65.
58 Alasdair Turner *et al.*, 'From isovists to visibility graphs: a methodology for the analysis of architectural space', *Environment and Planning B: Planning and Design*, 28 (2001), 103–21.
59 Bill Hillier and Julienne Hanson, *The Social Logic of Space* (Cambridge: Cambridge University Press, 1984).
60 'Environment', in this case, means the built or physical environment.
61 With VGA, Turner and colleagues (2001) sought to gain finer spatial differentiation metrics as an alternative to the comparatively large-grained and more importantly – manually generated – convex space discretisation of space.
62 It may be useful to conceptualise the immediate neighbourhood or reciprocally visible vertices as being able to be connected by a single straight line.
63 Detailed methods for constructing visual connectivity in Depthmap with graph set notation are found in Turner. Depthmap is a computer program that creates a base graph from an uploaded floorplan and is capable of generating isovists and VGA, among other forms of graph-based analyses Alasdair Turner, 'Depthmap: A program to perform visibility graph analysis', *Software* (2001).
64 Y. Choi, 'The morphology of exploration and encounter in museum layouts', *Environment and Planning B: Planning and Design*, 26 (1999), 241–50; Bill Hillier, 'Is architecture an *ars combinatoria*?', in *Space is the Machine: A Configurational Theory of Architecture* (Cambridge: Cambridge University Press, 1996), 216–61, https://discovery.ucl.ac.uk/id/eprint/3881/1/SITM.pdf; Alan Penn, Jake Desyllas and Laura Vaughan, 'The space of innovation: interaction and communication in the work environment', *Environment and Planning B: Planning and Design*, 26 (1999), 193–218, https://doi.org/10.1068/b4225; John Peponis *et al.*, 'Measuring the effects of layout upon visitors' spatial behaviors in open plan exhibition settings', *Environment and Planning B: Planning and Design*, 31, no. 3 (2004): 453–73, https://doi.org/10.1068/b3041; Kerstin Sailer, Andrew Budgen, Nathan Lonsdale, Alasdair Turner and Alan Penn, 'Comparative studies of offices pre and post – how changing spatial configurations affect organisational behaviours', (paper presented at the 7th International Space Syntax Symposium, Stockholm, Sweden, 2009); Kerstin Sailer and Alan Penn, 'The performance of space – exploring social and spatial phenomena of interaction patterns in an organisation' (paper presented at the International Architecture + Phenomenology Conference, Haifa, Israel, 2007); Margaret Serrato and Jean Wineman, 'Spatial and communication patterns in research and development facilities' (paper presented at the Proceedings of the Space Syntax Second International Symposium, Brasilia, 1999); Frieda D. Peatross, 'A syntactic study of control in restrictive settings: innovations in isovist methods', *Environment and Planning B: Planning and Design*, 28, no. 4 (2001), 529–44, https://doi.org/10.1068/b2708.
65 By 'generic', we mean spatial measures such as connectivity, integration, depth and so on, that are used across setting types and reflect probabilistic tendencies.
66 Unpublished seminar study, 2007. Colleagues included Professors Sonit Bafna and John Peponis, and classmates Yi Lu, Hui Cai, Bo Seo and Youngson Choi.
67 Lu and colleagues, 2009.
68 Ostensibly, TVi values would adjust according to the minimal and maximal number of heads of beds that one could simultaneously view; for example, if only four heads of bed were possible at one time, TVi values would range from 0–4.
69 Yi Lu *et al.*, 'Patient visibility and ICU mortality: a conceptual replication', *HERD*, 7, no. 2 (2014), 92–103.
70 Patient degree of illness is measured using various scoring systems; an APACHE II score >30 is a marker of severe illness. Yi, 'Patient visibility and ICU mortality'.
71 Michelle Ossmann and Sonit Bafna (unpublished work, 2010).
72 Agency for Healthcare Research and Quality, 'TeamSTEPPS®: National Implementation Research/Evidence Base', *TeamSTEPPS®: National Implementation Research/Evidence Base* (July 2015), https://www.ahrq.gov/teamstepps/evidence-base/teamstepps-research.html.

73 Dresser, 'The role of nursing surveillance in keeping patients safe'; Kelly and Vincent, 'The dimensions of nursing surveillance'; Agency for Healthcare Research and Quality, 'TeamSTEPPS®: National Implementation Research/Evidence Base'.

74 A full accounting of isovist connectivity with instructions for calculation is found in Michelle Ossmann, Sonit Bafna, Craig Zimring and David Murphy, 'Isovist connectivity: measuring the potential for concurrent targeted surveillance and general awareness', (paper presented at the 12th International Space Syntax Symposium, Beijing, China, 2019).

75 In addition to age, sex and ventilation days, we used illness severity (acuity) adjustment metrics, the sequential organ failure assessment (SOFA) scores day 1, and Charlson Comorbidity Index (CCI) scores.

76 The definitions, criteria and administrative coding for sepsis in this study are based on the 2001 recommendations. Mitchell M. Levy *et al.*, '2001 SCCM/ESICM/ACCP/ATS/SIS International Sepsis Definitions Conference', *Intensive Care Medicine*, 29, no. 4 (2003), 530–8, https://doi.org/10.1007/s00134-003-1662-x.

77 The rationale for selecting patients with a diagnosis of sepsis, DRG 870–2, has several origins. First, accepted acuity scales exist to quantify severity of illness; we used the SOFA score and the CCI. Second, the burdens associated with sepsis are enormous: treatment in the United States ran at an estimated $24 billion (6.2 per cent of total US hospital costs) in 2013. Anne B. Martin *et al.*, 'National Health spending in 2014: faster growth driven by coverage expansion and prescription drug spending', *Health Affairs*, 35, no. 1 (2017), 150–60, https://doi.org/10.1377/hlthaff.2015.1194. Sepsis is a leading cause of death and those who survive have an increased likelihood of long-term negative sequelae; Margaret Jean Hall *et al.*, 'Inpatient care for septicemia or sepsis: a challenge for patients and hospitals', *NCHS Data Brief*, no. 62 (June 2011), 1–8.

78 For specific architectural and interiors details by study ICU, see Michelle Ossmann, 'Exploring spatial risk: the impact of visibility on ICU mortality' (PhD, Georgia Tech, 2016).

79 At the time of the study, Emory University Health System was an academic tertiary referral centre with four hospital campuses, 12 ICUs, 173 critical care beds and more than 10,000 admissions annually.

80 W. Paul James and William Tatton-Brown, *Hospitals: Design and Development* (London: The Architectural Press, 1986).

81 Mahbub Rashid, 'A decade of adult intensive care unit design: a study of the physical design features of the best-practice examples', *Critical Care Nursing Quarterly*, 29, no. 4 (2006), 282–311.

82 Benedikt refers to the desired experience in space: 'to design environments not by the initial specification of real surfaces but by specification of the desired (potential) experience-in-space in the first place; that is by designing fields directly.' See Benedikt, 'To take hold of space: isovists and isovist fields', 63.

83 Patients who were transferred to other ICUs or who were readmitted to the ICU were excluded from analysis.

84 We examined a total number of 1,519 patient records; 1,385 (91 per cent) were eligible for inclusion.

85 For details on the Ward method for creating visibility groups, see Ossmann *et al.*, 'Isovist connectivity: measuring the potential for concurrent targeted surveillance and general awareness'.

86 We created visibility groups according to patient assignment to a low (n=877), medium (n=311) or high (n=197) isovist connectivity score room.

87 Severity of illness was measured with CCI and SOFA day 1.

88 For a full discussion section on the results of this study including limitations, refer to my doctoral dissertation, Ossmann, 'Exploring spatial risk: the impact of visibility on ICU mortality'.

89 Keith Hurst, 'UK ward design: patient dependency, nursing workload, staffing and quality – an observational study', *International Journal of Nursing Studies*, 45, no. 3 (September 2006), 370–81, https://doi.org/10.1016/j.ijnurstu.2006.09.007.

90 Joshi and colleagues replicated the method in Ossmann (2016) including step depth for isovist connectivity calculation and hierarchical clustering; ward method for creating low, medium and high isovist connectivity groups. Rutali Joshi, 'Impact of workstation enclosure and visual exposure on interruptions, collaboration and auditory environment during emergency physician handoffs' (PhD, Clemson, 2021).

References

Agency for Healthcare Research and Quality, 'TeamSTEPPS®: National Implementation Research/Evidence Base', *TeamSTEPPS®: National Implementation Research/Evidence Base* (July 2015), https://www.ahrq.gov/teamstepps/evidence-base/teamstepps-research.html.

Agency for Healthcare Research and Quality, 'Types of health care quality measures' (2015), https://www.ahrq.gov/talkingquality/measures/types.html.

Aiken, Linda H., 'Hospital nurse staffing and patient mortality, nurse burnout, and job dissatisfaction', *JAMA*, 288, no. 16 (23 October 2002), 1987–93, https://doi.org/10.1001/jama.288.16.1987.

Aiken, Linda H., *et al.*, 'Effects of hospital care environment on patient mortality and nurse outcomes', *The Journal of Nursing Administration*, 38, no. 5 (2008), 223–9, https://doi.org/10.1097/01.NNA.0000312773.42352.d7.

American Nurses Association, *ANAs Principles for Nurse Staffing* (Silver Spring MD: American Nurses Association, 2012).

Benedikt, Michael L., 'To take hold of space: isovists and isovist fields', *Environment and Planning B: Planning and Design*, 6 (2 January 1979), 47–65.

Benner, Patricia E., *From Novice to Expert: Excellence and Power in Clinical Nursing Practice* (Institute for Studies in Pragmaticism, 1984).

Carayon, Pascale, *et al.*, 'Work system design for patient safety: the SEIPS Model', *Quality and Safety in Health Care*, 15, no. suppl_1 (1 December 2006), 50–8, https://doi.org/10.1136/qshc.2005.015842.

Catrambone, Cathy, *et al.*, 'The design of adult acute care units in U.S. hospitals', *Journal of Nursing Scholarship*, 41, no. 1 (March 2009), 79–86, https://doi.org/10.1111/j.1547-5069.2009.01254.x.

Center for Medicare and Medicaid Services, 'Meaningful measure hub', *Meaningful Measures Framework* (10 September 2019), https://www.cms.gov/Medicare/Quality-Initiatives-Patient-Assessment-Instruments/QualityInitiativesGenInfo/MMF/General-info-Sub-Page.

Choi, Yoon Kyung, 'The morphology of exploration and encounter in museum layouts', *Environment and Planning B: Planning and Design*, 26 (1999), 241–50.

Clancy, Carolyn M., and David N. Tornberg, 'TeamSTEPPS: assuring optimal teamwork in clinical settings', *American Journal of Medical Quality*, 22, no. 3 (2007), 214–17, https://doi.org/10.1177/1062860607300616.

Clarke, Sean P., 'Failure to rescue: lessons from missed opportunity in care', *Nursing Inquiry*, 11, no. 2 (2004), 67–71.

Donabedian, Avedis, 'The quality of care', *JAMA*, 260, no. 12 (1988), 1743–8.

Dougherty, Cynthia M., 'Surveillance', in Gloria M. Bulecheck and Joanne C. McCloskey (eds), *Nursing Interventions: Effective Nursing Treatments* (3rd edition), (St Louis MO: Elsevier, 1999), 524–32.

Dresser, Susan, 'The role of nursing surveillance in keeping patients safe', *JONA: The Journal of Nursing Administration*, 42, no. 7/8 (2012), 361–8, doi:10.1097/nna.0b013e3182619377.

Dreyfus, Stuart E., 'The five-stage model of adult skill acquisition', *Bulletin of Science, Technology and Society*, 24, no. 3 (2004), 177–81, https://doi.org/10.1177/0270467604264992.

Gibson, James J., *The Ecological Approach to Visual Perception* (London: Lawrence Erlbaum Associates, 1986).

Griffiths, Peter, *et al.*, 'Nurse staffing, nursing assistants and hospital mortality: retrospective longitudinal cohort study', *BMJ Quality and Safety*, 28, no. 8 (2019), 609–17, https://doi.org/10.1136/bmjqs-2018-008043.

Gurses, Ayse P. and Pascale Carayon, 'Performance obstacles of intensive care nurses', *Nursing Research*, 56, no. 3 (2007), 185.

Hall, Kendall K., Demetrios N. Kyriacou, Jonathan A. Handler and James G. Adams, 'Impact of emergency department built environment on timeliness of physician assessment of patients with chest pain', *Environment and Behavior,* 40, no. 2 (2008), 233–48. https://doi.org/10.1177/0013916507311548.

Hall, Margaret Jean, *et al.*, 'Inpatient care for septicemia or sepsis: a challenge for patients and hospitals', *NCHS Data Brief*, no. 62 (June 2011), 1–8.

Heerwagen, Judith H., Kevin Kampschroer, Kevin M. Powell and Vivian Loftness, 'Collaborative knowledge work environments', *Building Research and Information*, 32, no. 6 (2004), 510–28.

Hendrich, Ann L., Marilyn P. Chow, Boguslaw A. Skierczynski and Zhenqiang Lu, 'A 36-hospital time and motion study: how do medical-surgical nurses spend their time?', *The Permanente Journal,* 12, no. 3 (2008), 25–34. https://doi.org/10.7812/tpp/08-021.

Hendrich, Ann L., Joy Fay and Amy K. Sorrells, 'Effects of acuity-adaptable rooms on flow of patients and delivery of care,' *American Journal of Critical Care*, 13, no. 1 (2004), 35–45, https://doi.org/10.4037/ajcc2004.13.1.35.

Henneman, Elizabeth A., Anna Gawlinski and Karen K. Giuliano, 'Surveillance: a strategy for improving patient safety in acute and critical care units', *Critical Care Nurse*, 32, no. 2 (31 March 2012), e9–18, https://doi.org/10.4037/ccn2012166.

Hillier, Bill, *Space is the Machine: A Configurational Theory of Architecture* (Cambridge: Cambridge University Press, 1996), https://discovery.ucl.ac.uk/id/eprint/3881/1/SITM.pdf.

Hillier, Bill, and Julienne Hanson, *The Social Logic of Space* (Cambridge: Cambridge University Press, 1984).

Holden, Richard J., *et al.*, 'SEIPS 2.0: a human factors framework for studying and improving the work of healthcare professionals and patients', *Ergonomics*, 56, no. 11 (2013), 1669–86, https://doi.org/10.1080/00140139.2013.838643.

Hurst, Keith, 'UK ward design: patient dependency, nursing workload, staffing and quality – an observational study', *International Journal of Nursing Studies*, 45, no. 3 (September 2006), 370–81, https://doi.org/10.1016/j.ijnurstu.2006.09.007.

Institute of Medicine, Ann Page (ed.), 'Keeping patients safe: transforming the work environment of nurses' (Washington DC: National Academies Press, 2004), doi:10.17226/10851.

James, Paul W., and William Tatton-Brown, *Hospitals: Design and Development* (London: The Architectural Press, 1986).

Joshi, Rutali, 'Impact of workstation enclosure and visual exposure on interruptions, collaboration and auditory environment during emergency physician handoffs' (PhD, Clemson, 2021).

Kalisch, Beatrice J., 'Missed nursing care: a qualitative study', *Journal of Nursing Care and Quality*, 21, no. 4 (2006), 306–13.

Kelly, Lesly, and Deborah Vincent, 'The dimensions of nursing surveillance: a concept analysis', *Journal of Advanced Nursing*, 67, 3 (March 2011), 652–61, https://doi.org/10.1111/j.1365-2648.2010.05525.x.

Kutney-Lee, Ann, Eileen T. Lake and Linda H. Aiken, 'Development of the hospital nurse surveillance capacity profile', *Research in Nursing and Health*, 32, no. 2 (April 2009), 217–28, https://doi.org/10.1002/nur.20316.

Lake, Eileen T., 'Development of the practice environment scale of the nursing work index', *Res Nurs Health*, 25, 3 (2002), 176–88.

Lake, Eileen T., *et al.*, 'A meta-analysis of the associations between the nurse work environment in hospitals and 4 sets of outcomes', *Medical Care*, 57, no. 5 (2019), 353–61, https://doi.org/10.1097/mlr.0000000000001109.

Lake, Eileen T., Kathryn A. Riman and Douglas M. Sloane, 'Improved work environments and staffing lead to less missed nursing care: a panel study', *Journal of Nursing Management*, 28, no. 8 (2020), 2157–65, https://doi.org/10.1111/jonm.12970.

Leaf, David E., Peter Homel and Phillip H. Factor, 'Relationship between ICU design and mortality', *Chest*, 137, no. 5 (May 2010), 1022–7, https://doi.org/10.1378/chest.09-1458.

Levy Mitchell M., *et al.*, '2001 SCCM/ESICM/ACCP/ATS/SIS International Sepsis Definitions Conference', *Intensive Care Medicine*, 29, no. 4 (2003), 530–8, https://doi.org/10.1007/s00134-003-1662-x.

Lu, Yi, 'Measuring the structure of visual fields in nursing units', *HERD*, 3, no. 2 (2010), 48–59.

Lu, Yi, John Peponis and Craig Zimring, 'Targeted visibility analysis in buildings: correlating targeted visibility analysis with distribution of people and their interactions within an intensive care unit', in Daniel Koch, Lars Marcus and Jesper Steen (eds), *Proceedings of the Seventh International Space Syntax Symposium* (Stockholm: Royal Institute of Technology, 2009), 68.1–68.10.

Lu, Yi, *et al.*, 'Patient visibility and ICU mortality: a conceptual replication', *HERD: Health Environments Research and Design Journal*, 7, no. 2 (2014), 92–103.

Martin, Anne B., *et al.*, 'National health spending in 2014: faster growth driven by coverage expansion and prescription drug spending', *Health Affairs*, 35, no. 1 (2017), 150–60, https://doi.org/10.1377/hlthaff.2015.1194.

Milhomme, Daniel, Johanne Gagnon and Kathleen Lechasseur, 'The clinical surveillance process as carried out by expert nurses in a critical care context: a theoretical explanation', *Intensive and Critical Care Nursing*, 44 (2018), 24–30, doi:10.1016/j.iccn.2017.07.010.

Mitchell, Pamela H., and Steven M. Shortell, 'Adverse outcomes and variations in organization of care delivery', *Medical Care*, 35, no. 11 (1997), 19–32, https://doi.org/10.1097/00005650-199711001-00003.

Mitchell, Pamela H., Jan Heinrich, Patricia Moritz and Ada Sue Hinshaw, 'Outcome measures and care delivery systems', *Medical Care*, 35, no. 11 (1997), 1–5, https://doi.org/10.1097/00005650-199711001-00001.

Needleman, Jack, *et al.*, 'Association of registered nurse and nursing support staffing with inpatient hospital mortality', *BMJ Quality and Safety*, 29, no. 1 (2020), 10–18, https://doi.org/10.1136/bmjqs-2018-009219.

Needleman, Jack, *et al.*, 'Nurse staffing and inpatient hospital mortality', *N Engl J Med*, 364, no. 11 (17 March 2011), 1037–45, https://doi.org/10.1056/nejmsa1001025.

Ossmann, Michelle, 'Exploring spatial risk: the impact of visibility on ICU mortality' (PhD, Georgia Tech, 2016).

Ossmann, Michelle, Sonit Bafna, Craig Zimring and David Murphy, 'Isovist connectivity: measuring the potential for concurrent targeted surveillance and general awareness', (paper presented at the 12th International Space Syntax Symposium, Beijing, China, 2019).

Peatross, Frieda D., 'A syntactic study of control in restrictive settings: innovations in isovist methods', *Environment and Planning B: Planning and Design*, 28, no. 4 (2001), 529–44, doi:10.1068/b2708.

Penn, Alan, Jake Desyllas and Laura Vaughan, 'The space of innovation: interaction and communication in the work environment', *Environment and Planning (B): Planning and Design*, 26, no. 2 (1999), 193–218., https://doi.org/10.1068/b4225

Peponis, John, *et al.*, 'Measuring the effects of layout upon visitors' spatial behaviors in open plan exhibition settings', *Environment and Planning B: Planning and Design*, 31, no. 3 (2004), 453–73, doi:10.1068/b3041.

Pfrimmer, Dale M., *et al.*, 'Surveillance', *Dimensions of Critical Care Nursing*, 36, no. 1 (2017), 45–52, doi:10.1097/dcc.0000000000000217.

Rashid, Mahbub, 'A decade of adult intensive care unit design: a study of the physical design features of the best-practice examples', *Critical Care Nursing Quarterly*, 29, no. 4 (2006), 282–311.

Rashid, Mahbub, 'Hospital design and face-to-face interaction among clinicians: a theoretical model', *HERD*, 2, no. 4 (2009), 62–84, https://doi.org/10.1177/193758670900200404.

Sailer, Kerstin, Andrew Budgen, Nathan Lonsdale, Alasdair Turner and Alan Penn, 'Comparative studies of offices pre and post – how changing spatial configurations affect organisational behaviours', (paper presented at the 7th International Space Syntax Symposium, Stockholm, Sweden, 2009).

Sailer, Kerstin, and Alan Penn, 'The performance of space – exploring social and spatial phenomena of interaction patterns in an organisation' (paper presented at the International Architecture + Phenomenology Conference, Haifa, Israel, 2007).

Serrato, Margaret, and Jean Wineman, 'Spatial and communication patterns in research and development facilities', (paper presented at the Proceedings of the Space Syntax Second International Symposium, Brasilia, 1999).

Shekelle, Paul G., 'Nurse-patient ratios as a patient safety strategy: a systematic review', *Annals of Internal Medicine* 158, 5, Pt 2 (5 March 2013), 404–9, https://doi.org/10.7326/0003-4819-158-5-201303051-00007.

Tandy, C., 'The isovist method of landscape survey', in H. C. Murray (ed.), *Symposium: Methods of Landscape Analysis* (London: Landscape Research Group, 1967), 9–10.

The Joint Commission, 'Sentinel event', *Patient Safety Topics* (2021), https://www.jointcommission.org/resources/patient-safety-topics/sentinel-event/.

Thompson, Dan R., *et al.*, 'Guidelines for intensive care unit design', *Critical Care Medicine*, 40, no. 5 (May 2012), 1586–600, doi:10.1097/ccm.0b013e3182413bb2.

Trzpuc, Stefnee J., and Caren S. Martin, 'Application of space syntax theory in the study of medical-surgical nursing units in urban hospitals', *HERD*, 4, 1 (2010), 34–55, https://doi.org/10.1177/193758671000400104.

Tucker, Anita L., *et al.*, 'Front-line staff perspectives on opportunities for improving the safety and efficiency of hospital work systems', *Health Services Research*, 43, no. 5 (2008), 1807–29, https://doi.org/10.1111/j.1475-6773.2008.00868.x.

Turner, Alasdair, 'Depthmap: a program to perform visibility graph analysis', *Software* (2001).

Turner, Alasdair, *et al.*, 'From isovists to visibility graphs: a methodology for the analysis of architectural space', *Environment and Planning B: Planning and Design*, 28 (2001), 103–21.

Ulrich, Roger, Craig Zimring, Xuemei Zhu, Jennifer DuBose, Hyun-Bo Seo, Young-Seon Choi, Xiaobo Quan and Anjali Joseph, 'A review of the research literature on evidence-based healthcare design', *HERD: Health Environments Research and Design Journal*, 1, no. 3 (2008), 61–125.

Wedel, S., *et al.*, 'Guidelines for intensive care unit design: guidelines/practice parameters committee of the American College of Critical Care Medicine, Society of Critical Care Medicine', *Critical Care Medicine*, 23, no. 3 (March 1995), 582–8.

Chapter 3 Table
Introduction

The chapter theme ‘table’ conveys a focus on design and the complex formal and informal group functioning that is an essential but little-understood dimension of hospital-based care. The chapter, authored by Rosica Pachilova and Kerstin Sailer, advocates for a view of nurses as knowledge workers, with the implication that nurse travel on wards should be understood in terms based on its capacity to support team communication and collaboration, in sharp conceptual departure from a focus on the shortness of travel distances. To this end, they describe the development of the Spaces for Communication Index (SCI), which assesses accumulated visibility, and therefore opportunity for encounter, along high-use trajectories of inpatient wards. Pachilova and Sailer have found that the SCI correlates with higher measures of healthcare quality, indicating a potential link from layout to quality via design-based support for team communication.

In her response essay, Upali Nanda picks up the theme of balancing concern for efficiency, visibility to patients and what she calls ‘human scripts’. In addition to describing practice-based field research on inpatient wards, Nanda notes the potential value of a metric such as the SCI in assessing the special status of the inpatient ward corridor as a hub of communication, awareness and movement.

Together, the chapter and essay provide a fresh perspective on teamwork in hospitals, especially in terms of recognising the value of nurses talking.

Working together in healthcare space

Rosica Pachilova and Kerstin Sailer

Healthcare work is increasingly complex and relies on a multitude of different professionals – doctors, nurses, anaesthetists, phlebotomists, physiotherapists, porters, cleaners, caterers and many others – all working together to provide care and support for patients. During the course of a four-day hospital stay, the care for one patient may involve as many as 50 different healthcare providers.

It may seem a truism to argue that working together is inherent to today's healthcare environment, yet what we mean by 'working together' is not a settled matter (see Figure 3.1). An editorial in the *British Medical Journal* notes the difference between simply working side-by-side and actually working together,[1] noting that existing collaborative practices are rudimentary and hindered by multiple barriers, including obstinate medical traditions and rigid role identities such that 'the tales that nurses and doctors each tell about the other when they are outside work and "among friends" suggest that there is still some way to go'.[2]

Different communities working together has been highlighted as a key factor to organisational learning:

> To foster working, learning, and innovating, an organization … needs to reconceive of itself as a community-of-communities, acknowledging in the process the many noncanonical communities in its midst. It must see beyond its canonical abstractions of practice to the rich, full-blooded activities themselves. And it must legitimize and support the myriad enacting activities perpetrated by its different members.[3]

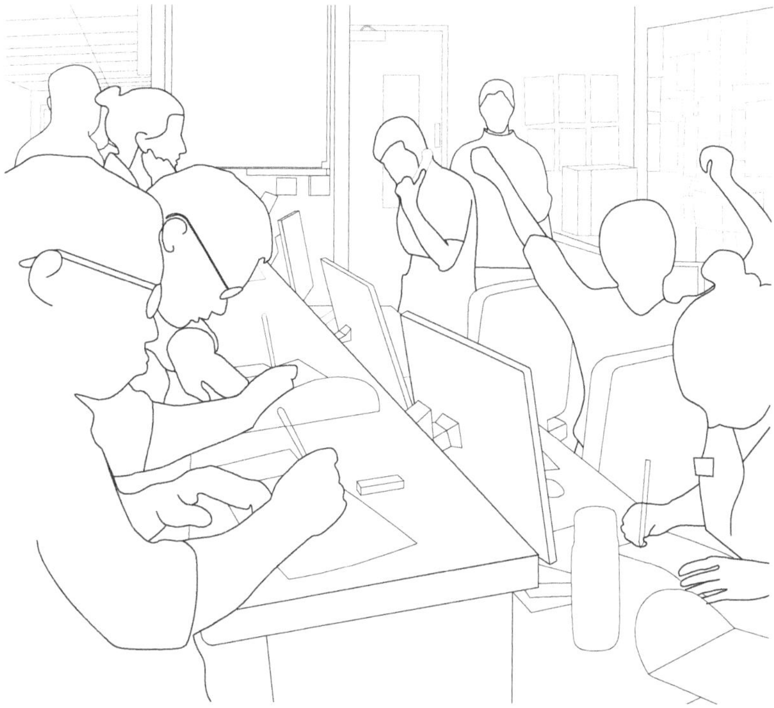

3.1 Working side-by-side or teamwork in a nurse station? Drawn by Victor Carrillo and Daniel Rios, 2021.

What Brown and Duguid argue here is that an organisation wanting to develop and thrive must listen to its diverse communities and their members. At the bottom of their argument lies the insight that learning happens day to day and on the ground in everyday practices and builds on sense-making, interpretations and adaptations of routines and actions. Communities of practice form essential bottom-up building blocks within organisations and the whole organisation is in essence a 'community-of-communities'.

Considering communities in healthcare work is nothing new. Writing from the perspective of research for design, Rashid proposes that the different professionals working in healthcare are part of overlapping communities: each community engages in its own particular knowledge domain, their community of practice, as well as being part of communities of interest, where individuals from different knowledge domains come together to perform a specific task, such as in a multidisciplinary team that forms around a critically ill patient.[4]

The theory of overlapping communities of practice is all well and good, but how does collaboration work in practice? How can we develop a view of healthcare work that is rooted in its social, interactive nature? And what role does the spatial layout of hospitals play in orchestrating how people come together and communicate?

In this chapter, we interpret the history of hospital work in tandem with that of analytical approaches to hospital design. Many narratives on these themes amount to stories focusing on individual effort and separated professions, and this atomistic view of hospital work has lent itself to a focus on the individual worker (e.g., their efficiency and work practices), rather than developing concepts and measures on teamwork and collective processes and outcomes. We aim to extend these approaches with a social perspective on care, arguing that communication is a key component of healthcare and that health professionals are, in many cases, knowledge workers that require healthcare layouts better suited to the nature of their work in the twenty-first century.

Healthcare work and the division of labour: a brief history

Throughout most of history, nurses, doctors and other formal and informal practitioners learned their art through oral traditions passed from generation to generation, observing others caring for the sick and often gaining insight through processes of trial and error. Care was provided mostly in one's own home, where family members and friends acted as caregivers. Outside of the home, it was usually nuns and monks who provided care for the sick in European hospitals, often sought only by those who had no family members or by those whose work took them away from their homes.[5] Between 1100 and 1300, early modern medical schools were founded in Europe in university cities such as Paris, Bologna and Oxford. Medieval doctors analysed symptoms, made diagnoses and either administered medications or prescribed a diet, rest, sleep, exercise or baths. Surgeons could treat fractures and dislocations, repair hernias and perform amputations and a handful of other operations. With the advent of early modern medicine, formalisation and standardisation of practice began to transform the medical profession into an institution. Meanwhile, childbirth was left to midwives, as a care type that still relied heavily on folklore and tradition.[6] As a consequence of this differentiation between the two professions, doctors and nurses worked in silos. Up until the late nineteenth century when Florence Nightingale (see Figure 3.2) began a movement to recognise nursing as a profession in its own right, nurses were positioned as servants to doctors, and their contribution to

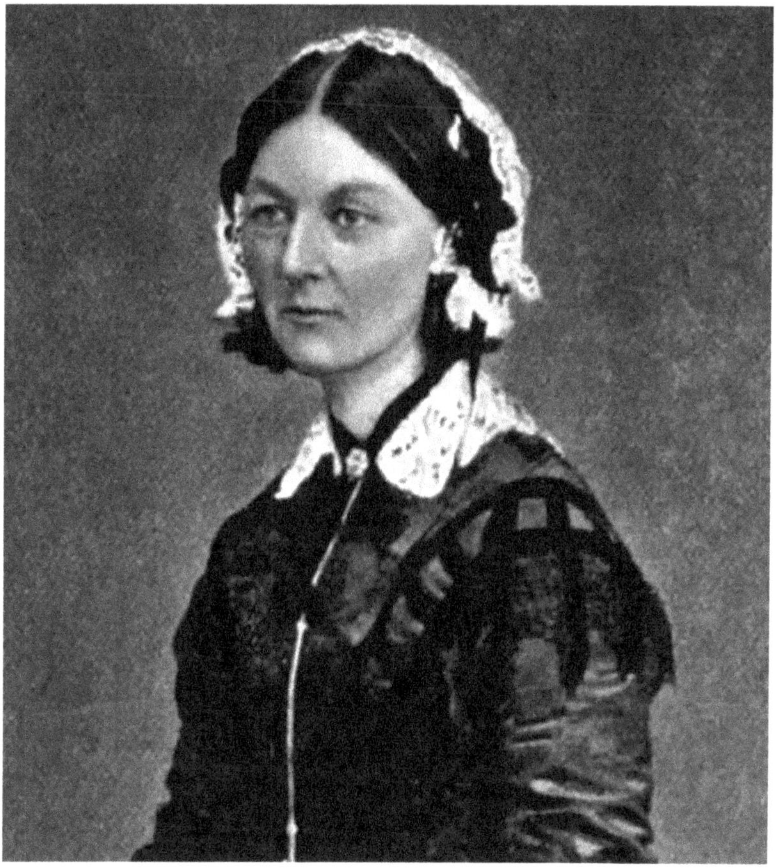

3.2 *Florence Nightingale*. Image credit: Jess Sweeney through Wikimedia Commons.

patient care was deemed a mere extension of the doctor's knowledge and competence. To that end, this view of the history of medicine is very much conceived through the eyes of doctors as the dominant medical profession, leaving little space for alternative readings, such as from nurses, those providing care in communities, or even from the perspective of sufferers.[7]

Healthcare has long been characterised by an overt and significant division of labour, similar to other domains of work. In *The Wealth of Nations*, Adam Smith argues that increases in productive powers are due to the division of labour.[8] In their discussion of the history of the organisation of work, Kranzberg and Hannan[9] go even further, contending that the division of labour was at the heart of human evolution and development as our prehistoric ancestors began inventing tools.

Individual proficiency or skill in specific tasks gave rise to early forms of specialisation (e.g., hunting versus gathering) and from there to the formation of professions (e.g., potters, textile makers, farmers, metal workers and so on). The by-product of division of labour, a surplus of goods, was responsible for the way in which human civilisations grew and prospered, leading to even more sophisticated ways of dividing labour, not just by proficiency, but by gender, class and age. It was the French sociologist Emile Durkheim who pointed out that there is more to the division of labour than pure efficiency. Specifically, the fundamental role of the division of labour is a principle that creates societal bonds and establishes social solidarities between people who rely on each other to survive.[10] This social function, Durkheim added, plays an ethical role and ultimately makes society possible in the first place. When we think of professional communities in healthcare settings, it is worth keeping both elements of the division of labour in mind: how it creates efficiency and how it acts as social 'glue'.

It is not controversial to argue that the nursing profession contributes to the social glue in healthcare environments, possibly more than any other profession. Although extensive writing addresses the role of nursing and the character of nurse work, we might say that the history of nursing work is still being written and is very much in flux as we continually reflect on the role of nurses and how that role evolves. The nurse has been variously defined as the assistant who supports the powers of the doctor, as the creator of the ideal conditions for patient healing,[11] and as an extension of the patient who bridges gaps created by the patient's reduced capabilities.[12] In focusing on teamwork and solidarity, we would like to follow a recent redefinition of nurse work[13] that sees nurses as healthcare mediators. When evaluating the actual work activities of nurses and defining bundles of nurse practices (e.g., managing the work of others, managing multiple agendas, maintaining records, rounding), the role of the nurse emerges as an intermediary, as the professional who moderates the relationship between healthcare systems and different practitioners and thus constitutes contexts of care.

But before we follow this line of thought further, it is worth looking back in history to two major developments in how healthcare workspace was defined and shaped. First, the work of Florence Nightingale shaped nursing as a profession, though it arguably also reduced nursing to concerns with ventilation, sanitation and surveillance. Second, time-motion studies evaluated the number of movements and amount of time that it took to achieve a certain task with the aim of task optimisation – this approach become a popular way to bring work processes and ward layouts together into a single analytical framework. We will show how these two developments of nurse work are intertwined inside a paradigm of efficiency.

Florence Nightingale: the cure of open air

The history of nursing is often conflated with the story of Florence Nightingale and her efforts to improve the care of the wounded during the Crimean War. She established the principles under which women could provide comfort and care in what had been a male-dominated hospital environment under the role of 'nurse'. Nightingale also established nursing as a secular profession through her role in the Nightingale School of Nursing at St Thomas' Hospital in London, which educated professional nurses in what was the first such secular institution, opening in 1860. Student nurses received classes in theory coupled with clinical experience on hospital wards.

The story of Florence Nightingale famously began when she learned that the mortality rate of British troops during the Crimean War was 41 per cent. Soldiers were dying from disease rather than from their injuries because of the poor conditions in field hospitals. Nightingale believed that dirt was the cause of disease and embarked on a campaign to thoroughly scrub the soldiers' barracks and hospital wards and let in sunshine and fresh air; and these tactics decreased the number of deaths dramatically. Mary Seacole, a lesser-known female pioneer of nursing, was a British-Jamaican contemporary of Nightingale who worked with the same principles to fight a cholera epidemic in Panama in the 1850s. She reported a similar set of tactics in her autobiography: 'By my directions, doors and shutters were open, fires were lighted, and every effort was made to ventilate the place.'[14]

But it was Nightingale who left the much clearer mark in history. In addition to her work in nursing as such, she also laid foundations for modern evidence-based practice. Nightingale was a pioneer in the graphical representation of data. At a time when research reports were only beginning to include tables, Nightingale was using bar charts and pie charts that were colour coded to highlight her points (see Figure 3.3). She was keen not only to get the science right but to also make it comprehensible to lay people. One recommendation that she made was for the creation of a statistical department to track rates of disease and mortality and to identify problems so that they could be dealt with promptly.

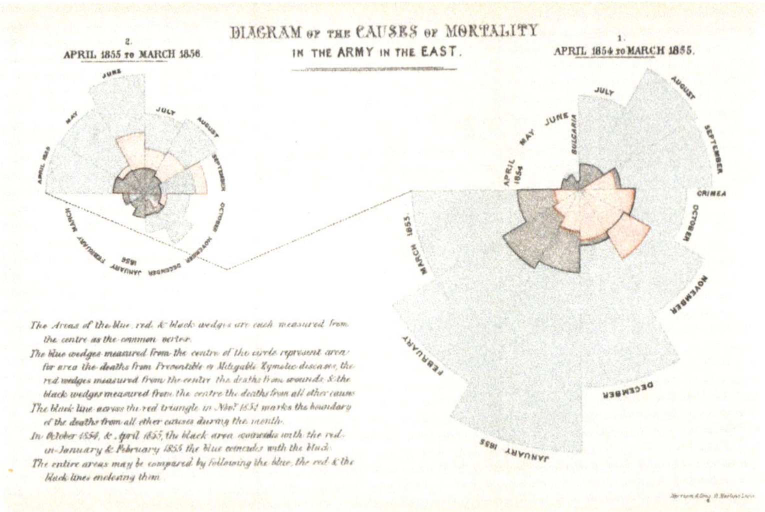

3.3 Florence Nightingale's diagram of the causes of mortality in the army, 1820–1910. Image credit: Wikimedia Commons.

Nightingale's contributions to nursing were certainly groundbreaking. Much of our practice in ventilation, sanitation and the importance of handwashing and hygiene are owed to her. The open-plan ward typology named after her (see Figure 3.4) was almost a by-product of allowing light and air to penetrate wards, as otherwise cross-ventilation and airflow (before the advent of mechanical ventilation) would not have been possible. With Nightingale's principles of open air came a high degree of visibility between carers and patients, building on earlier hospital layout examples.[15]

Critically reflecting on a Nightingalian approach from today's point of view, we cannot help but notice how much the cure of open air radically reduces the definition of nurse work to tasks in maintaining cleanliness. It set the scene for a scientific and rule-driven treatment of patients that increased patient safety and gave newly trained nurses clear guidelines to follow. Yet, it also roots nursing practice firmly in efficient work organisation principles that, while important in an industrialising society, have revealed their shortcomings in the twenty-first century. The next section shows how Nightingale's valuation of efficiency became an explicit planning principle in the twentieth century and assumed dominance over the discourse on how healthcare ought to be organised.

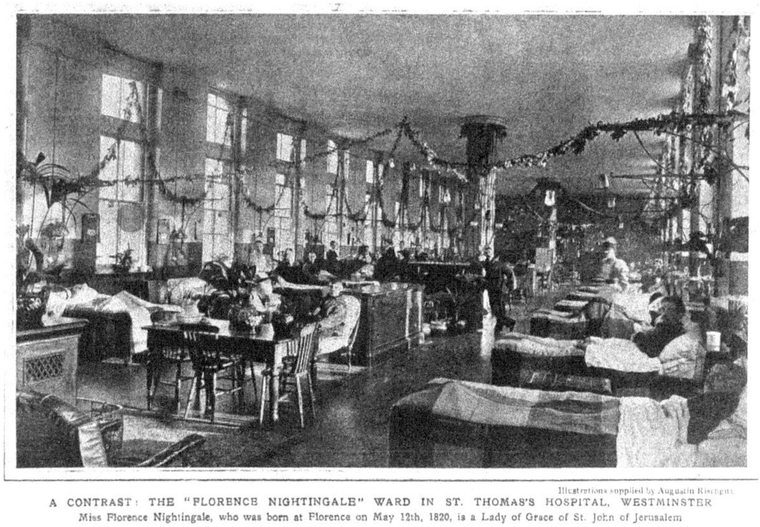
Illustrations supplied by Augustin Rischgitz
A CONTRAST: THE "FLORENCE NIGHTINGALE" WARD IN ST. THOMAS'S HOSPITAL, WESTMINSTER
Miss Florence Nightingale, who was born at Florence on May 12th, 1820, is a Lady of Grace of St. John of Jerusalem

3.4 A Nightingale ward at St Thomas's Hospital, 1900. Image credit: Augustine Rischgitz via Wikimedia Commons.

Time-motion studies: the rule of efficiency

The early twentieth century witnessed the end of the second industrial revolution, which gave rise to vast corporations in the United States. As new entities, these organisations initially operated inefficiently, wasting a lot of material resources. The way that jobs were done varied wildly from person to person – some people were proficient, others less so. Around this time, Frederick Taylor, a mechanical engineer in a steel company, developed a special interest in the study of industrial processes focused on the global issue of inefficiency.[16] In Taylor's view, the task of factory management was to determine the best way for the worker to do the job, to provide the proper tools and training and to supply incentives for good performance. In his studies, Taylor undertook detailed observations of workers using a stopwatch to determine the time required to accomplish specific tasks. With unnecessary tasks eliminated, the worker, following a machine-like routine and focusing on time, became far more productive. On the first day using Taylor's new method, the number of products that the workers in a factory were able to transport almost tripled. This method was later expanded by Taylor's disciples, Frank and Lilian Gilbreth, who focused on motion. The motion study method sought to make processes more efficient by reducing the physical movements involved. These two techniques, time studies and motion

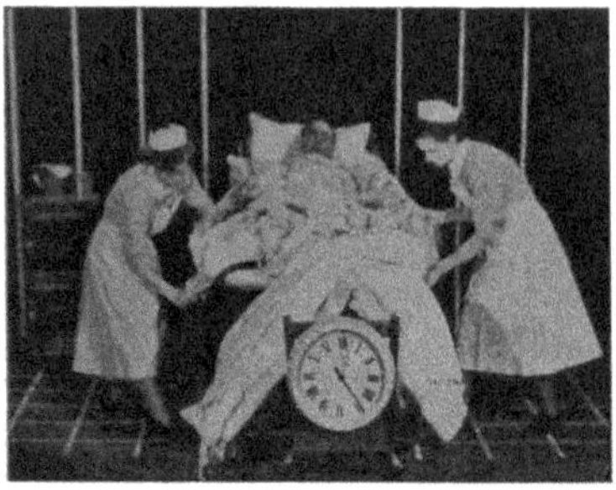

Fig. 7. The space needed to make a bed with the patient in it

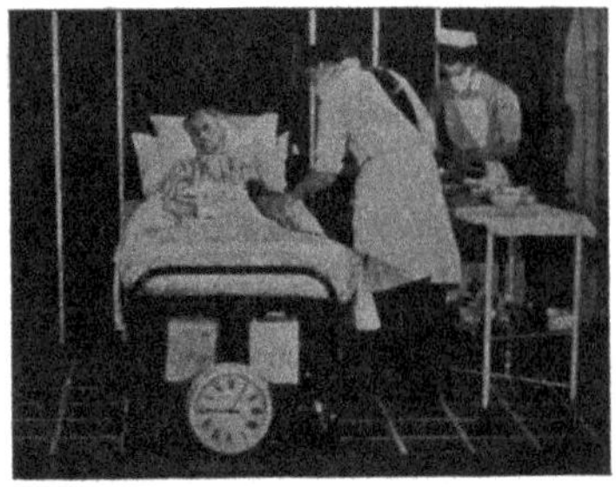

Fig. 8. The space needed to set up an intravenous transfusion at the bedside

3.5a and 3.5b Studies in space required for nurses to make a bed (left) and set up an intravenous transfusion (right).

studies, became integrated into a widely accepted method in scientific management referred to as time-motion studies.

Since then, time-motion studies have been broadly adopted by researchers in the field of healthcare management (see Figures 3.5a and 3.5b) and have become a focus of attention due to interest in clinical workflow-related factors. Architecturally inspired research in this tradition focused not only on efficiency but also on ward typologies, aiming to establish general insights on how to best design wards.

After World War Two, the Nuffield Foundation undertook an interdisciplinary approach to systematically investigate the design of hospitals. The research team published the seminal report *Studies in the Functions and Design of Hospitals*,[17] where they discussed the configuration of patient wards and the optimisation of nurses' work areas based on observations of healthcare worker movement, gluing a plan to a corkboard and marking worker movements with strings wrapped around pins (see Figure 3.6). The data gathered through these diagrams led to the conclusion that the utility room should be close to the bed area. Optimal room arrangements were inferred based on the underlying premises that the less nurses walked the better and that reduced walking would convert into increased time for patient care and improved patient safety and outcomes.

This line of reasoning was advanced with more systematic accounts of ward-based walking distances. Such an example is the Yale Traffic Index, developed by Thompson and Goldin[18] in the 1970s, which followed a Taylorist approach. The aim of the index was to compare general medical and nursing units for functional efficiency with the suggestion that the best performing layout would minimise walking distances between functional areas of a ward, such as patient beds and nurse

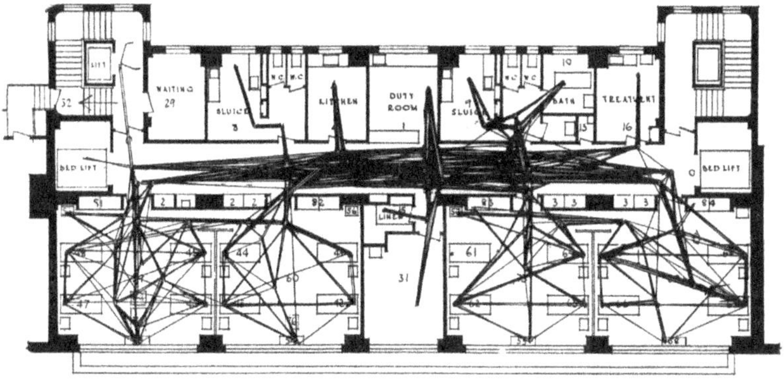

Fig. 5. The pattern of movement of a nurse in training, during a complete tour of duty in a ward unit in the National Hospital, Queen Square

3.6 Mapping student nurse travel, 1955. By kind permission of the Trustees of University College London Hospitals NHS Foundation Trust.

stations. From such information, it could be inferred which areas of the inpatient ward should be placed in close proximity to each other. After following healthcare providers for six months in four nursing units in Yale-New Haven Hospital, Thompson and Goldin identified 16 areas on a typical nursing ward that were most frequently used, including patient rooms, nurse stations, utility rooms, elevator lobbies, medication closets and pantries. They recorded the number of trips between each pair of areas, which they referred to as 'links', and identified the 14 most frequently traversed links. They then multiplied key links by their associated distance measures, then added together these products and divided the sum by the number of patient beds on the ward (to account for ward size). The resulting Yale Traffic Index combined constant values for estimating trip frequency together with values for trip distances that could be plugged in for different layouts. This index could thus be used to make comparative evaluations of units with similar facilities (or programmatic elements) but different floorplan configurations. The smaller the index value, the shorter the estimated total travel distance over a 24-hour period and thus the more efficient the layout. The method was applied to 30 inpatient units and it was found that wards with redundant circulation schemes, such as double-corridor units or circular plans, were more efficient than double-loaded single-corridor plans.

This strict focus on ward efficiency by means of minimising walking distances has remained dominant in the discourse on healthcare architecture. It is worth noting how the quest for a generalisable simple answer on how best to spatially arrange a ward ended in recommendations for layout typologies, specifically radial plans or double-corridor plans. Such recommendations are easily actionable by architects, yet they rest problematically on three overly simplified ideas about nurse work. First, equating quality care practices with least time spent walking paints a reductionist picture of healthcare work, very much in line with the Taylorist notion that good work means maximum efficiency and minimal waste. Second, efficiency is measured on a per-individual basis in this case, as walking (or other locomotion for workers with mobility impairments) is an activity that every healthcare worker engages in separately. Third, there is a presumption of a single and apparently correct way of performing duties, which is to follow the routines as modelled, again closely aligned with the ethos of Taylor and his 'scientific' management.

However, one cannot streamline knowledge work in the same way that one can automate car manufacturing or optimise tracking requisitions. Knowledge work is ever-changing, dynamic and autonomous. It centres on problem solving and requires both convergent and divergent thinking to answer questions that arise in daily work.[19] What often looks like slacking at work, such as long conversations in the break room, tearoom or café, are often activities that are conducive to building professional and friendship relationships, to sharing ideas and knowledge that can contribute to innovations, as is often expected of knowledge workers. Building professional and friendly relations and collaboration are often important aspects of knowledge work. However, recognising the knowledge dimension of nurse work and establishing collaborative practices between doctors and nurses has been a significant challenge facing healthcare organisations since hospitals still operate through hierarchies, silos and very strong professional cultures that can be an obstacle to implementing a high-performing work environment.

Collaborative practice and communication: healthcare as knowledge work

At the heart of any collaborative practice is the process of good communication. For instance, in a study of an intensive care unit (ICU), it was shown that verbal miscommunication between nurses and doctors was responsible for 37 per cent of all errors.[20] Failed communication between poorly coordinated teams was identified as a major contributor to errors.[21] In addition, collaboration between doctors and nurses has been found to increase team members' awareness of each other's knowledge and skills, leading to continued improvement in decision making.[22]

Nevertheless, collaborative practices between doctors and nurses are not so straightforward, given an entire history of separation between the two professions characterised by long-held hierarchies and differences in esteem placed on doctors and nurses, with doctors (historically men) making the 'important' decisions, while nurses (historically women) tending to the personal environment of the patient. Yet change is on the horizon. With the growing sophistication of medical care, more educated nurses have been prepared to care for and treat patients with increasingly complex conditions and needs. Several important social changes have further altered the doctor-nurse relationship in the past 50 years, including an increase in the number of female doctors and the generally improved status of women in society and the workplace.[23]

It is easy to think of doctors as knowledge workers, yet on mediating the role of nurses and their role in sharing and distributing information, it is clear that this is also knowledge work. Nurses are no longer mere direct-care providers. They are problem solvers and decision makers, working from high levels of expertise, education and experience. Nurse work depends heavily on sharing knowledge and expertise, for which communication is crucial. In this sense, we can read the division of labour in healthcare as Durkheimian, as a means of creating social glue, over and above improving efficiency.

A focus on collaborative practice makes healthcare work no different from other forms of knowledge-intensive work. Vertical communication, extensive collaboration across disciplinary boundaries, knowledge sharing and networked forms of organisation are readily accepted as the norm for white-collar, office-based, service-oriented and technology-driven work in the twenty-first century. The same is true for healthcare environments.

How collaborative practices unfold in everyday healthcare activities and, interestingly, where exactly they unfold, is our next concern. To examine this, we draw on Goffman's dramaturgical theory that uses the metaphor of the backstage and the front stage, where actions are performed for an audience.[24] In contrast with the formal activities of the front stage, backstage activities are more informal, allowing the individual to relax the role played on the front stage and prepare to re-emerge onto the front stage in role again.

Goffman's theory was used by Lewin and Reeves[25] to study teamwork in a hospital ward. Lewin's and Reeves' observations led them to interpret front stage activities as those when members of the care team were performing their roles in front of patients and families, such as during rounding. Rounding is, of course, intended to facilitate and maintain interprofessional teamwork, including via doctor-nurse communication. However, both doctors and nurses noted that, with few exceptions, nurses rarely joined the medical rounds, let alone communicated with doctors during rounds. Their findings suggested that inter-professional work was more *ad hoc* and opportunistic and was generally more feasible as a backstage activity. Corridor conversations, in particular, were conducive to overcoming the inhibition of cross-professional communication that was observed on the front stage. The backstage interactions were short, task-orientated and prone to interruption.

Spaces for knowledge-intensive collaborative healthcare work need to accommodate but also support informal and unplanned encounters in the same manner that office work relies on chance meetings, serendipity and 'water-cooler moments'.[26]

From designing for individual work to designing for teamwork

The previous section highlighted the importance of the knowledge worker in healthcare settings, but it also identified the role of the physical environment for communication and knowledge exchange between different team members. The following section will dive into hospital settings and how design influences the movement and interaction patterns of healthcare workers.

Lewin and Reeves[27] highlight the importance of the main ward corridor as a 'backstage' space for supporting informal and unplanned conversations between persons with different professional roles, with the richness and rapid feedback of in-person communication helping to reduce communication errors.[28] The corridor has also been referred to as a neutral zone that is not 'owned' by any particular discipline.[29] In this neutral zone, nurses, doctors, physical therapists and other healthcare professionals interact spontaneously and opportunistically. In these spaces, not only do higher-status professionals such as doctors, express more uncertainty about diagnosis and treatment options, but they also seek out, listen to and act on views and information from other professional staff.

Formal communications in hospitals are often expressed with certainty, while in corridor conversations there is greater room for contingencies,[30] breeches of decorum and suspension of the usual professional hierarchies. It is the corridor that allows the occupational therapist to interrupt the doctor or the peer support worker to interject with an emotional response that would never appear in a front-stage setting. Corridors also tend to mix the various user types of a given setting.[31] Instead of considering corridors a waste of space,[32] they should be seen as constituting a greater circulatory system while affording specific behaviours, in the same way that urban streets are part of a hierarchy of connecting routes as well as loci of human activity. The corridor can be designed for its multiple purposes, especially recognising the important role that it plays in providing ample opportunities for nurse-doctor communication.

The importance of the main corridor has also been demonstrated by space syntax researchers looking into the importance of the whole spatial configuration of the ward for communication, and in particular how different spatial elements such as corridors and rooms are put together in a spatial network that affects movement and encounter patterns. Existing studies have investigated and demonstrated the effect of openness, visibility and proximity of spaces on communication and thus provided a detailed and accurate description of the layout. For example, Choudhary and her colleagues[33] developed a space syntax model to predict the effect of different hospital ward layouts on the random and unplanned movement generated by nurses, which was affected by the spatial and visual properties of their assigned sub-areas. This study showed that sub-areas with larger viewsheds and shorter path lengths resulted in fewer trips to patient rooms because of better visibility. Another study investigated the effect of ward configuration on movement and developed a measure called 'targeted visibility',[34] which calculated the visibility towards a number of pre-selected visual targets, in this case patient beds. The study showed that more nurses could be expected in areas with higher targeted visibility to patients; while doctors more often occupied areas with higher overall visibility, often found in corridors and intersections. A different study[35] demonstrated that when assigned to a low visibility room, the most acute patients had significantly higher ICU mortality rates. Targeted visibility measures suggested as potential mechanisms associated with these results include 'field of view' and 'distance', with outcomes such as time at the bedside, actual patient observation and response times. Other studies found that patients were seen sooner when placed in a room without doors and closer to the physician workstations[36] and nurses visited their patients more frequently when their room assignments were more integrated.[37] Still, other studies, such as that by Nanda and colleagues,[38] demonstrate how movement is driven by use frequencies and distances between key programmatic elements.

These findings illustrate that the configuration of the ward layout is important for communication. However, the measures described above are based on the idea that individuals move around and position themselves visually in relation either to the patient or the overall unit layout. The measures do not specifically take into consideration the interdisciplinary and team-based nature of inpatient work. Further, while the aforementioned measures point to interesting aspects of the physical environment that affect movement and communication, they remain difficult to translate into design decisions or even discussions with design teams.

The importance of visibility for communication in office-based workplaces has been demonstrated by multiple studies.[39] In healthcare environments, studies have shown that bringing team workers closer together and increasing openness among them increased communication between them[40] and made it easier to coordinate care and thus improve patient experience.[41] Separating staff facilities from patient areas also had a positive effect on communication between staff members, as they could discuss confidential information with other colleagues without being overheard by patients.[42]

Given these research foundations, which suggested a social logic of nurse work that is related to spatial visibility, we developed a new single measure called the 'Spaces for Communication Index' (otherwise 'SCI'), which draws on ideas from both the Yale Traffic Index and Choudhary's model. We incorporated the aggregative concept from the Yale Traffic Index. However, instead of embedding efficiency as a concept expressed by distances walked by individuals, we aimed to focus on the work of the healthcare team. Rather than measuring space efficiency in the form of minimising distances, the SCI measures space effectiveness in the form of maximising communication opportunities related to teamwork, a crucial provision of good healthcare. We also aimed to develop a metric that could be applied with ease to ward design. Details on our approach and the development of the metric are reported elsewhere.[43] In the next section, we briefly describe the SCI and its basis in the recognition that the provision of healthcare requires knowledge workers who operate in a twenty-first-century organisation that functions as a network of professionals communicating easily with each other.

Designing for teamwork: the SCI

People are not static, and are even less so in healthcare environments, so it is unsurprising that doctors and nurses have quite dynamic movement patterns. They can go back and forth multiple times per hour from one key location to another. Depending on the specific configuration of a ward, those key functional areas can be positioned in spaces with higher or lower visibility. Moreover, the corridors and spaces that connect them also provide different levels of visibility. A healthcare worker can go between two spaces with low visibility and on the way pass through a space with high visibility. In terms of nurse visibility to one another, it is not just the visibility levels of key locations that matter, but also how much visibility gets 'accumulated' along their typical paths of travel. We found that the higher the accumulated visibility along the work path of a healthcare worker, the more they actually communicated with others.[44] This statistically significant relationship showed that accumulated visibility can be used as a valid proxy for actual communication behaviour. The SCI indicated the potential for communication opportunities that arise from the visibility properties of the layout and walking patterns of healthcare providers. However, we focused SCI on capturing support for teamwork rather than support for the work behaviour of individuals.

Movement pattern data from six inpatient units were used to develop the SCI. Across all six cases, a total of 71 nursing staff were followed by an observer for an average of 40 minutes each while they went about their work. The information was used to identify the most frequently traversed paths by nurses between key areas in a hospital ward which included:

1. patient beds – nursing station;
2. patient beds – medicine room;
3. patient beds – patient beds; and
4. nursing station – medicine room.

These accounted for nearly 90 per cent of all movement paths of the observed nurses in the six cases, which varied in type and size of the ward, staffing patterns and bed capacity. The way that the SCI was calculated was very similar to the Yale Traffic Index. However, instead of the physical distances between key locations, we took the average visibility of the paths that link key areas and multiplied this by the number of times a path must be traversed derived from the observations in the six case studies (see Figure 3.7). The resulting numbers were added together and the total was divided by the number of patient beds to normalise for the size of each ward.

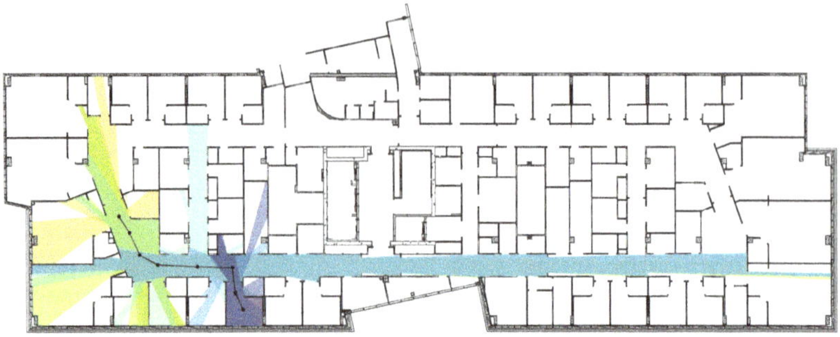

3.7 Concept diagram showing the principle of accumulated visual exposure for a typical nurse task path. For the SCI, the sum of exposure for task paths are multiplied by estimated task frequency. Concept diagram by Victor Carrillo and Daniel Rios, 2021.

We calculated the SCI for a larger sample of 31 different wards in the United Kingdom and found that the unit with the best quality of care[45] was the one that provided healthcare workers with maximum opportunities for communication as measured by accumulated visibility, the underlying principle of the SCI. The larger in size the sum of the viewsheds along the path that linked one key function to another, the higher the chances of bumping into another healthcare worker and having an informal, quick conversation, where important patient information could be exchanged. Wards with a larger SCI value – typically with larger viewsheds on key paths – were more likely to have outstanding healthcare quality as rated by the UK Care Quality Commission than wards with smaller SCI values. The findings of this research also make sense intuitively: spaces with larger viewsheds allow for frequent and easy exchanges among healthcare workers. Even social chit chat, such as exchanging smiles or greetings, can contribute to a productive workplace environment. We also calculated the Yale Traffic Index for these wards; however, this efficiency-based measure seemed to have less of a direct relationship to healthcare quality in our sample.

Towards a generalisation of SCI

After the SCI was developed, we conducted further explorations on how designers could use the tool to evaluate their ward layouts. In particular, we were curious to see how generalisable the SCI is and if it can be specifically applied to more enclosed environments, such as wards with only single-patient rooms. Our initial database contained mostly wards with four-bed to six-bed bays, but single-patient rooms are generally preferred by patients and family members because they provide privacy and quiet, which helps patients to heal more quickly.[46] They also enable family members to stay overnight. Single-patient rooms work better when it comes to infection control and preventing the spread of infectious diseases, which, post-COVID, is an even more important requirement for hospitals. On the other hand, single-patient rooms are less preferred by some nurses because they act as a barrier to surveillance, communication and socialisation and, in the case of newer nurses, restrict their learning opportunities.

To test the generalisability of the SCI, we selected four additional case studies, drawing on inpatient wards in four US hospitals designed and shared with us by HKS Architects. The wards varied in area from a minimum of 1,130 m^2 to a maximum of 2,000 m^2 and in number of patient rooms from 28 to 36. All units followed a consistent layout format, with patient rooms located along the perimeter of the building to provide views and natural daylight to patients, support facilities in the core and corridors surrounding the support areas serving each room. All cases have two or more team nursing stations in key locations to create proximity and visibility to clusters of patient rooms (see Figure 3.8).

In this sample of 100 per cent single-patient room wards, the ward with the greatest SCI values is a racetrack unit with four corridors crossing between the two longest corridors (case D, see Figure 3.8). The other three units had lower, very similar SCI values. They had layouts with more geometrically complex floorplates and multiple corridors. A spatial analysis of the visual connectivity[47] of these cases indicated the higher visibility conditions in the highest SCI case was driven by generous views wherever orthogonal corridors crossed. In the other three cases, only one similarly high-visibility intersection between the two longest main corridors was identified. Further, in these cases, the width of the corridor was narrower compared to the high-SCI case, resulting in less visual openness along key paths.

The four case studies had a lower SCI score compared to the initial database of hospitals, which included multi-patient rooms and open bays. This was anticipated because the average ward visibility levels in the fully single-patient room environments are lower. That said, creating larger viewsheds along critical nurse paths can be achieved by design in

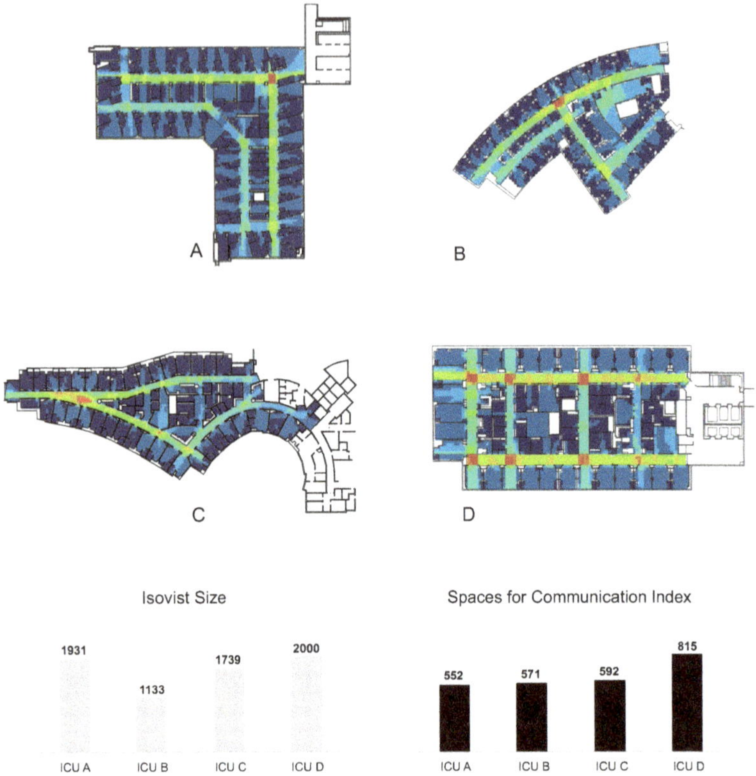

3.8 Visual connectivity graphs for 100 per cent single-room wards, with SCI values listed. Image by Rosica Pachilova, 2019.

any ward typology. As for fully single-patient room wards, there were four such cases in our initial database (see Figure 3.9). Two of these wards had high SCI indices and good ratings of healthcare quality, while two had lower SCI and were rated as requiring improvement. The ward that had the highest SCI rating in the initial database, and was ranked for outstanding quality of care, was a radial ward with 100 per cent single-patient rooms. What likely made the SCI score higher than expected for an enclosed environment was a large circular space in the middle of the ward that connected all patient rooms. This space provided high-visibility levels to nurses and doctors who had to pass through it on their way from one key area to another. The SCI can provide insight on layout and support for caregiver collaboration, but we are emphatically not advocating for any specific layout typology, radial or otherwise. Creating larger viewsheds along key paths can be achieved by design in any ward typology.

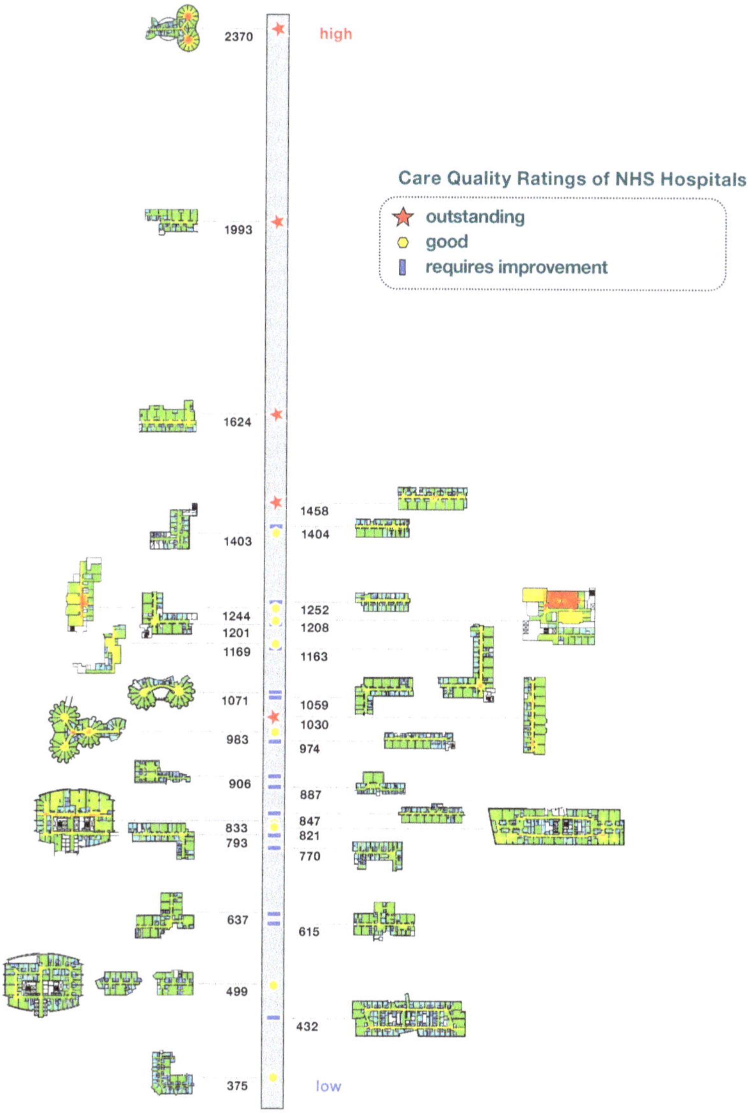

3.9 The SCI of UK inpatient wards, with National Health Service Care Quality Ratings, and wards with 100 per cent single-patient rooms called out. Image by Rosica Pachilova, 2019.

The SCI enables designers and healthcare operators to run a speculative model and, based on its results, begin to lead informed conversations with designers and healthcare professionals about layout and teamwork. In the following section, we suggest some general principles for layout that are likely to raise the SCI in almost any ward layout. However, we first wish to describe some limitations of our study to date.

The development of our method in UK hospitals involved empirical observations of the wards in action, studies of communication patterns and empirical work on the socio-spatial realities that shaped work processes and the collaborative practices of doctors and nurses. The extension of the method to US-based examples does not include a similar baseline assessment of workflows, frequently traversed paths, staffing ratios or patient satisfaction data, among other things. We look forward to conducting continued empirical research in these areas.

Design interventions for more communication opportunities

Teamwork in healthcare requires communication opportunities, and we have argued that these are built into the spatial fabric of wards. We therefore conducted investigations to understand what layout attributes affect the SCI and what interventions designers and healthcare planners can make that could lead to more communication opportunities. Below, we look closely at two wards from the initial database, both of which were from the same hospital but had different healthcare quality ratings. The first, an ICU ward, had better care quality and consisted mostly of four-bed bays and some single-patient rooms; it had an SCI score of 821. The second, a general nursing ward, had a worse care quality rating and a layout with more single rooms and some bays. This ward had a lower SCI score of 432.

We tested three different interventions on the layout of the wards. In the first option, we increased the width of the main corridor (the most connected area) by 50 cm. In the second option, we created large, open spaces at key locations to increase the levels of visibility at those locations. In the final option, we changed the nurse station model and thus the movement associated with nurse assignments. The ICU ward uses a decentralised nurse station model where every two inpatient room or a four-bed patient bay has a nurse station that allows the nurse to stay closer to the patient. The general nursing ward has two centralised nurse stations located symmetrically on both sides of the ward which allows nurses to stay closer to each other. To study the effects of nursing model difference, we flipped the nursing models in each case study. The ICU ward had a centralised nursing station located in the corridor while the nursing ward layout had decentralised nursing stations in each patient room or bay. An illustration of the three different changes in the nursing ward is shown in Figure 3.10.

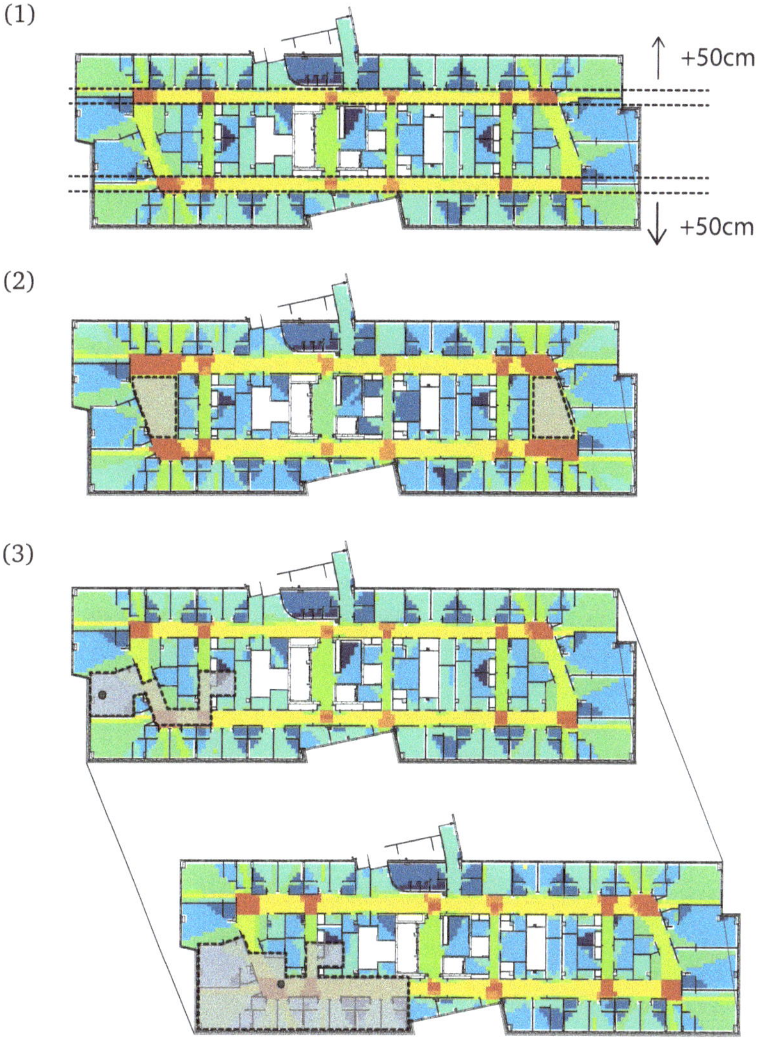

3.10 Layout strategies tested for effect on SCI. (1) Increased corridor width by 50 cm; (2) Enlarged open space at corridor crossings with high visual connectivity; and (3) Change nurse assignment from centralised (bottom) to decentralised (top) nurse-station model and vice versa. Image by Rosica Pachilova, 2019, redrawn by Victor Carrillo and Daniel Rios, 2021.

By making the corridor wider in the first design alteration, the SCI increased by 7 per cent in the ICU ward and by 19 per cent in the nursing ward. Creating larger open spaces in key locations increased the SCI by 10 per cent in the ICU and by 43 per cent in the nursing ward. Finally, changing the nurse assignment from a decentralised to a centralised nursing station model in the ICU increased the SCI by 2 per cent while implementing decentralised stations and associated travel patterns in the nursing ward decreased the SCI by 23 per cent.

These experiments illustrate design principles that have been shown to support communication through layout. Namely:

1. Creating large, open spaces at key functional locations drives up visual connectivity and thus spaces for communication.
2. Widening corridors, even to a moderate degree, has a similar effect, although of a smaller magnitude in these particular examples.
3. In addition, centralised nursing station models tend to create more movement and opportunities for interaction than the decentralised nursing station models.

These design strategies – open spaces, wider hallways and team spaces for nurses – are directly applicable when it comes to the design of hospital wards, but still draw on some principles revealed though SCI analysis. Our research suggests that to maximise communication opportunities, wards should have at least one large open space at a key location in a way that links increased visibility levels with 'attractor' functions, or key areas that are frequently visited by nurses. The number of these large open spaces and their size and function are driven by the specific project, client and design goals. Intuitively, it makes sense for these spaces to accommodate teamwork areas including the nursing station, but they may also be enriched with facilities for doctors and other healthcare professionals to promote cross-disciplinary teamwork.

Working together in healthcare space

This chapter briefly reviewed the history of the doctor and nursing professions, following the move from siloed practices towards a culture of working together, with a specific focus on how the concept of nurse work has fed into principles for the design of hospital wards. Nurses were initially viewed as servants to doctors until Florence Nightingale began a movement to professionalise nurse work. More recently, nurses have come to be seen as moderators of the relationship between healthcare systems and different practitioners, and the importance of collaborative practices and communication for the delivery of safe and quality healthcare is acknowledged. The first spatial element recognised as important to the team was the corridor, the significance and design of which is still too often neglected. In providing a neutral zone and a backstage, in Goffman's sense of the term, the unit corridor affords a space for different healthcare professionals to communicate spontaneously and opportunistically across hierarchies and professional silos.

As we regard nurses as knowledge workers who require a workplace layout that supports communication and teamwork, we developed the SCI to focus on supporting the healthcare team, not just the individual. Using the SCI, we demonstrated that wards with larger accumulated viewsheds on main paths between key functional areas were rated more highly on measures of healthcare quality. Larger viewsheds appear to allow for frequent and easy informal conversations among healthcare workers. What the SCI enables designers and healthcare planners to do is to run a speculative model and, based on its results, to begin a focused and informed discussion about the layout design. Our measure can be translated easily to design decisions, including strategies about strategic open spaces, corridor widths and nurse station models. With increases in the SCI, we anticipate increased opportunities for chance encounters.

Our aim is to help bridge the gap between academia and industry and, with our knowledge and research tools, contribute to the design of future hospital wards by engaging with architects and healthcare planners. We advocate for a view of nurses as knowledge workers whose day-to-day tasks, alongside others, involve problem solving, reasoning, critical thinking, decision making, creativity and learning. Future hospital designs should acknowledge that an effective hospital ward design encourages teamwork and the provision of integrated care, supporting communication and exchange between doctors and nurses.

Response Essay: Spatial intelligence to support a team-of-teams ecosystem – relevance and need in practice

Upali Nanda

'Communities of practice form essential bottom-up building blocks within organisations, and the whole organisation is in essence a "community-of-communities".' With this statement, Pachilova and Sailer capture the essence of modern-day healthcare in describing the complex, overlapped and ultimately social entities that comprise healthcare organisations. As average longevity increases at a population level, so too does the complexity of providing healthcare. In the past few years, team-based care has emerged as one of the key shifts necessary to address this complexity. Nowhere is the team-based approach as important as in the inpatient unit itself, where an ecosystem of care is enacted every single day.

The design of the inpatient unit is arguably one of the most important components of the design of any hospital. The care model of a facility drives the unit design, and the key drivers usually call for care that is patient-centred, team-based and value-driven. Unfortunately, the team-based conversation, by and large, has been too focused on efficiency, and has thus been reduced to over-simplified debates, such as between decentralised versus centralised nurse stations. This false dichotomy can be problematic.

At M. D. Anderson Cancer Center, for example, the research and design teams at HKS Architects found that a fully centralised model posed challenges to efficiencies, while a fully decentralised model created challenges to peer-to-peer communication. After studying both models at M. D. Anderson, we developed a hybrid system with a range of spaces, including a central team station, decentralised stations directly outside the patient rooms and touch-down stations for teams on the move. M. D. Anderson also invested in spaces by the patient bedside, where much of the focused work and patient coordination happens.[48]

Our work with M. D. Anderson revealed a tiered concept for the inpatient unit workplace focused on transfer of knowledge and coordination of care. These included:

1. the patient bedside (tier 1);
2. the decentralised workstation right outside the patient room where individual heads-down work and small consultations take place (tier 2);
3. larger team stations, with a team room for focused interaction, through activities such as teaching, safety huddles and the like, or a conference room for scheduled meetings (tier 3); and
4. quick-stop or touchdown stations for teams on the move (tier 4).

This tiered approach with full digital integration (virtual work) is a hybrid one, which is neither centralised nor decentralised, and navigates between the digital and physical world to support a team-of-teams work ecosystem, responsive to the dynamic work conditions in health.

Research suggests that compared with teams in other industries, healthcare teams have more dynamic work conditions, frequent changes in team membership, various specialised members and interprofessional and multidisciplinary cultures.[49] Our research looked at communication data in the RN ecosystem, showing survey-based self-report from oncology nurses on communication frequency with others. It supports Pachilova and Sailer's points about the role of the nurse as an intermediary, as the professional who moderates the relationship between healthcare systems and different practitioners and thus constitutes contexts of care. A hybrid approach in a tiered model conceptualises the designed environment for such a role.

In Promedica Medical Center (see Figure 3.11), the tiered approach emphasised team-based care by increasing alcove spaces and prioritising

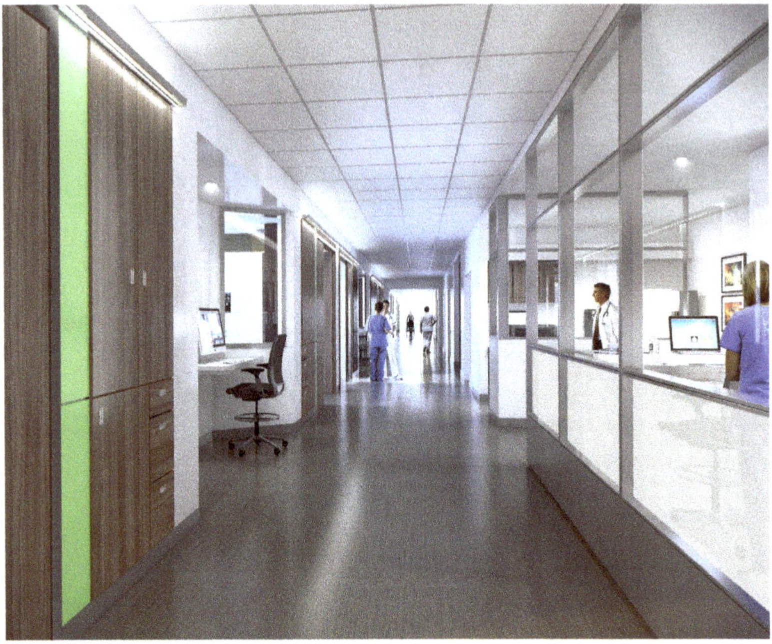

3.11 Promedica inpatient tower design after using spatial analytics to reduce hide-away spaces, increase peer-peer and patient-provider visibility, and reduce wasted walking, 2020. Copyright HKS Architects.

mobile workstations. The corridor is used not as a travel space that separates but rather as a collaboration conduit. A year into occupancy, a post-occupancy diagnostic will be conducted to allow an objective assessment of the efficacy of a hybrid approach to team-based care. The Promedica post-occupancy study will also be a test of how the tiered approach works.

In studying plan function, the focus has traditionally been on efficiency, *vis-à-vis* a more holistic effectiveness. Further, plans are often studied without focus on the essential behavioural layer that contributes to health outcomes. While designing a new unit, old behavioural and operational patterns from existing facilities can be inadvertently carried forward, an inheritance that can pose challenges to the success of a new facility.

Design demands diagnostics that layer observed, reported and spatial insights

In our work we deploy a tool called the 'design diagnostic', to study the relationship between facility design, human experience and organisational efficiency; to understand the current state, and to provide inputs to the design of the future state. All of this happens *during* the course of a project. Typically, design diagnostics are used when a unit is moving to a

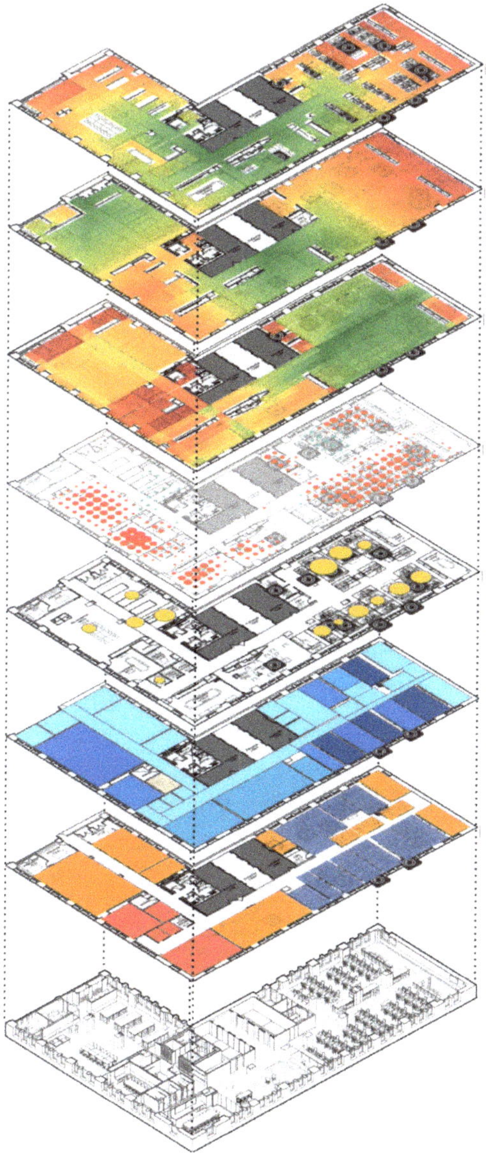

3.12 A layered mapping tool to link spatial and human analytics from Soleimani, Nanda and Augustine, 2020. Copyright HKS Architects.

new environment, whether renovated or greenfield, and they are akin to a diagnostic that a physician would employ to understand a health issue before prescribing a treatment.[50] Design diagnostics are meant to provide a layer of objective information to complement the subjective insights from typical user group meetings and to bridge the disconnect between what people say and what people do within a clearly defined physical environment context. This design diagnostic is a composite tool (see Figure 3.12) that has an on-site and an off-site component, with elements that can be conducted either on-site or off-site, using three types of data:

1. Observed – Insights about the space, and users' interaction with the space in its 'natural' or everyday condition. These are collected via behaviour mapping, shadowing and photo-essays on site.
2. Reported – Insights from users about their space, processes and experience. These are collected via survey or interviews.
3. Spatial – Insights from plans to assess key affordances of the space and how they compare to other similar units. These are collected via simple benchmarking (comparing sizes and areas) and parametric analysis of proximity between key rooms, visibility between key areas and walking distances between key areas. Walking distances are simulated based on the observed data from field research.

Currently, our team is working on a prototype tool called 'Onion', which layers spatial and behavioural insights to take a more nuanced approach to correlating the spatial and the human to advance health and systemic outcomes.[51]

Linking design to outcomes

In the field of applied design research, the ability to correlate health outcomes to design affordances, including spatial parameters, is paramount. A variable such as walking distance can be linked to both human and organisational outcomes, as they are impacted by relatively simple, straightforward dimensions of inpatient units.[52]

In a study of ICU plans, researchers found that nurse-rated visual contact with peers could be explained by integration of key work zones, while time at the patient bedside was correlated to the local shape properties of the plan in terms of the link between patient rooms and nurse stations.[53] The analysis of key components like adjacencies, walking distances, integration and visibility, are becoming mainstream, although there remains a struggle with the lack of industry benchmarks on which measures are most important and what their thresholds for success are. Regarding the former concern, Pachilova and Sailer are correct in critiquing the focus on operational efficiency that is based on the legacy of time-motion studies.

In previous work, we have argued that simple adjacencies and proximities are not enough; the human scripts must be understood. In an early study on Promedica Health System using the design diagnostic, we found that core issues in the workspace related to:

1. waste and variability in walking;
2. limited point-of-use access to supplies;
3. large distances travelled for minor tasks; and
4. low visibility and connectivity.

We also found that the corridor was used as a workspace/communication hub, which prompted our development of the tiered approach and the articulation of the corridor discussed above.[54] However, at the time, we did not find a spatial metric that could help assess the value of the corridor towards its intended function as a communication hub or spine in the context of the human scripts of movement.

SCI: from intention to application

A key piece missing from the puzzle of relevant spatial analytics is the ability to assess, objectively, healthcare plans for potential to promote communication and camaraderie. The SCI fills this crucial gap in literature. The concept of accumulated visibility along the work path of a healthcare worker and its relationship to level of communication is a key contribution of this work. Taking the average visibility of a space and multiplying this by the number of times a path must be traversed allows a nuanced, context-responsive approach that brings together human scripts and spatial affordances. It also allows us to shift our current understanding of hospitals as units of efficiency to dynamic knowledge ecosystems.

The next step would be to use this measure extensively in a wide range of projects and create a robust database that could provide that elusive goal for our industry: a benchmark against which we can measure success that has generalisability, as well as enough flexibility for contextual application. Clients at architecture firms should be offered the opportunity to donate plans and encouraged to share evaluations and outcomes. Internal tools such as the ones discussed here should be infused with this metric as well, so that it can continue to be validated.

While staff-to-staff communication is an important factor in the design of hospital units, there are at least two other established parameters involved in the design: visibility in patient units; and walking distances. The latter, in particular, has the potential to conflict with the SCI measure, since the more a person walks in a unit and the more spaces are traversed, the higher the total value. A future study can investigate the conflict between these parameters and the ways in which a hospital can be designed for all three of them. This is an interesting optimisation question with implications for generative design.

Eventually, the architecture industry will need agile tools with robust foundations that can meet the needs of the rapid pace of projects. Given the complexity of our industry, a layered approach where the interactions between spatial and human metrics are constantly assessed and optimised will be vital. It is my hope that bringing industry and academia together in tool development, tool testing and contribution to non-proprietary databases will allow us to move the needle in the profession and allow spaces to be a primary tool in creating the social glue that Pachilova and Sailer so articulately describe.

Acknowledgements

For their very helpful feedback and comments, the author wishes to thank Kate Renner, AIA, Senior medical planner at HKS Architects, and Babak Soleimani, PhD, Design researcher and data analyst at HKS Architects.

Notes

1 Celia Davies, 'Getting health professionals to work together: There's more to collaboration than simply working side by side', *BMJ,* 320, no. 7241 (2000), 1021–2, https://doi.org/10.1136/bmj.320.7241.1021.
2 Davies, 'Getting health professionals to work together', 1022.
3 John Seely Brown and Paul Duguid, 'Organizational learning and communities of practice: toward a unified view of working, learning, and innovation', *Organization Science,* 2, no. 1 (1991), 40–57. The quote is from page 53.
4 Mahbub Rashid, 'Hospital design and face-to-face interaction among clinicians: a theoretical model', *HERD*, 2, no. 4 (2009), 62–84, https://doi.org/10.1177/193758670900200404.
5 Karen J. Egenes, 'History of nursing', in Gayle Roux and Judith Halstead (eds), *Issues and Trends in Nursing: Essential Knowledge for Today and Tomorrow* (Burlington MA: Jones and Bartlett Publishers, 2009), 1–27.
6 'History of medicine – Hellenistic and Roman medicine', in *Encyclopaedia Britannica*, https://www.britannica.com/science/history-of-medicine/Hellenistic-and-Roman-medicine#ref35655 (accessed 14 January 2021).
7 The idea of the 'sufferer' puts the ill person, their feelings, identity and their bodily as well as emotional experiences at the centre of the discussion. Referring to them as patients would already presume a hospitalised and medicalised gaze. For more information, see Roy Porter,

'The patient's view', *Theory and Society,* 14, no. 2 (1985), 175–98, https://doi.org/10.1007/bf00157532.

8 Adam Smith, *An Inquiry into the Nature and Causes of the Wealth of Nations* (London: W. Strahan and T. Cadell, 1776).

9 Melvin Kranzberg and Michael T. Hannan, 'History of the organization of work', in *Encyclopaedia Britannica*, https://www.britannica.com/topic/history-of-work-organization-648000 (accessed 14 January 2021).

10 Emile Durkheim., *The Division of Labor in Society* (New York: The Free Press, 1893).

11 This is a Nightingale-inspired definition and one that many nurses subscribe to today.

12 This line of argument proposes that nurses aim to restore completeness, wholeness and independence in a patient, and while the patient is ill, nurses take over the role of their eyes, ears, limbs, etc. See Virginia Henderson, 'The nature of nursing', *The American Journal of Nursing,* 64, no. 8 (1964), 62–8.

13 Davina Allen, 'Re-reading nursing and re-writing practice: towards an empirically based reformulation of the nursing mandate', *Nursing Inquiry,* 11, no. 4 (2004), 271–83, https://doi.org/10.1111/j.1440-1800.2004.00234.x.

14 Jenni Murray, *A History of Britain in 21 Women: A Personal Selection* (New York: Simon & Schuster, 2016).

15 For a more complete overview of a history of hospital buildings, see Chapter 4 ('Re-Formation') in Thomas A. Markus, *Buildings and Power: Freedom and Control in the Origin of Modern Building Types* (London: Routledge, 1993).

16 Frederick W. Taylor, *The Principles of Scientific Management* (New York: Harper & Brothers, 1911), https://archive.org/details/principlesofscie00taylrich/mode/2up.

17 Nuffield Provincial Hospitals Trust and the University of Bristol, *Studies in the Functions and Design of Hospitals* (1955), https://www.nuffieldtrust.org.uk/files/2017-01/functions-and-design-of-hospitals-web-final.pdf (accessed 14 January 2021).

18 Thompson and Goldin identified 16 areas on a typical nursing ward and recorded the number of trips between each pair of areas, which were referred to as 'links'. They identified the 14 most frequently traversed links that were considered the prime determinants of unit efficiency. The relative trip frequencies of these links were multiplied by distance measures, the result being referred to as the 'Yale Traffic Index'. See John D. Thompson and Grace Goldin, *The Hospital: A Social and Architectural History* (New Haven CT and London: Yale University Press, 1975).

19 Peter Drucker, *Landmarks of Tomorrow* (New York: Harper, 1959).

20 Yoel Donchin, Daniel Gopher, Miriam Olin, Yehuda Badihi, Michal B. Biesky, Charles L. Sprung, Ruven Pizov and Shamay Cotev, 'A look into the nature and causes of human errors in the intensive care unit', *Critical Care Medicine,* 23, no. 2 (1995), 294–300, https://doi.org/10.1097/00003246-199502000-00015.

21 Peter I. Buerhaus, 'Follow-up conversation with Lucian Leape on errors and adverse events in health care', *Nursing Outlook,* 49, no. 2 (2001), 73–7, doi:10.1067/mno.2001.114404.

22 Caryn Christensen and James R. Larson, 'Collaborative medical decision making', *Medical Decision Making,* 13, no. 4 (1993), 339–46, https://doi.org/10.1177/0272989x9301300410.

23 Christensen and Larson, 'Collaborative medical decision making'.

24 Erving Goffman, *The Presentation of Self in Everyday Life* (Harmondsworth: Penguin Books, 1959).

25 Simon Lewin and Scott Reeves, 'Enacting "team" and "teamwork": Using Goffman's theory of impression management to illuminate interprofessional practice on hospital wards', *Social Science and Medicine,* 72, no. 10 (2011), 1595–602, https://doi.org/10.1016/j.socscimed.2011.03.037.

26 A recent article in the *Harvard Business Review* even goes as far as to suggest that 'collisionable hours' (i.e., the degree to which colleagues bump into each other in unplanned ways) is important in office design. See Ben Waber, Jennifer Magnolfi and Greg Lindsay, 'Workspaces that move people', *Harvard Business Review,* 92, no. 10 (2014), 68–77.

27 Lewin and Reeves, 'Enacting "team" and "teamwork"', 1595–602.

28 Jane Carthey, 'Reinterpreting the hospital corridor: "wasted space" or essential for quality multidisciplinary clinical care?', *HERD,* 2, no. 1 (2008), 17–29, https://doi.org/10.1177/193758670800200103.

29 Franklin Becker, 'Nursing unit design and communication patterns: what is "real" work?', *HERD,* 1, no. 1 (2007), 58–62, https://doi.org/10.1177/193758670700100115.

30 Rick Iedema, Debbi Long, Katherine Carroll, Maree Stenglin and Jeffrey Braithwaite, 'Corridor work: how liminal space becomes a resource for handling complexities of multi-disciplinary health care' (paper presented at APROS 11: Asia-Pacific Researchers in Organization Studies 11th International Colloquium, Melbourne, Australia, 2005).

31 This is the focus of Chapter 4 of this book, authored by Sonit Bafna and Julie Zook.

32 Carthey, 'Reinterpreting the hospital corridor', 17–29.

33 Ruchi Choudhary, Sonit Bafna, Yeonsook Heo, Ann Hendrich and Marilyn Chow, 'A predictive model for computing the influence of space layouts on nurses' movement in hospital units', *Journal of Building Performance Simulation,* 3, no. 3 (2010), 171–84, https://doi.org/10.1080/19401490903174280.

34 Yi Lu, John Peponis and Craig Zimring, 'Targeted visibility analysis in buildings: correlating targeted visibility analysis with distribution of people and their interactions within an intensive care unit', in Daniel Koch, Lars Marcus and Jesper Steen (eds), *Proceedings of the Seventh International Space Syntax Symposium* (Stockholm: Royal Institute of Technology, 2009), 68.1–68.10.

35 Yi Lu and Craig Zimring, 'Can intensive care staff see their patients? An improved visibility analysis methodology', *Environment and Behavior,* 44, no. 6 (2011), 861–76, https://doi.org/10.1177/0013916511405314.

36 Kendall K. Hall, Demetrios N. Kyriacou, Jonathan A. Handler and James G. Adams, 'Impact of emergency department built environment on timeliness of physician assessment of patients with chest pain', *Environment and Behavior,* 40, no. 2 (2008), 233–48, https://doi.org/10.1177/0013916507311548.

37 Ann Hendrich, Marilyn P. Chow, Boguslaw A. Skierczynski and Zhenqiang Lu, 'A 36-hospital time and motion study: how do medical-surgical nurses spend their time?', *The Permanente Journal* (2008), 25–34; Upali Nanda, Sipra Pati and Adeleh Nejati, 'Field research and parametric analysis in a medical-surgical unit', *HERD*, 8, no. 4, (2015), 41–57.https://doi.org/10.1177/1937586715577370.

38 Nanda, Pati and Nejati, 'Field research and parametric analysis in a medical-surgical unit'.

39 In office-based workplaces, the effect of visibility on communication among co-workers is established by a collection of scholarly work throughout the decades. In 1992, Backhouse and Drew showed that immediate visibility between colleagues resulted in communication events, often arising from one person walking past someone else's desk. See Alan Backhouse and Peter Drew, 'The design implications of social interaction in a workplace setting', *Environment and Planning B: Planning and Design*, 19 (1992), 573–84. Swedish researchers confirmed that communication events anchored to desks based on mutual visibility between staff; see Henrik Markhede and Daniel Koch, 'Positioning analysis: social structures in configurative modelling' (paper presented at the 6th International Space Syntax Symposium, Istanbul, June 2007) 12–15; Jesper Steen, 'Spatial and social configurations in offices' (paper presented at the 7th International Space Syntax Symposium, Stockholm, Stockholm, 2009). Most recently, a larger sample of offices was investigated, highlighting that areas with higher overall strategic visibility attract more communication events; see Petros Koutsolampros, Kerstin Sailer, Tasos Varoudis and Rosie Haslem, 'Dissecting visibility graph analysis: the metrics and their role in understanding workplace human behaviour', in *12th International Space Syntax Symposium* (Beijing: Beijing Jiaotong University, 2019), 1–24 (paper no. 191).

40 Rosica Pachilova and Kerstin Sailer, 'Evidence-based design: the effect of hospital layouts on the caregiver-patient interfaces' (paper presented at 2nd European Conference on Design 4 Health, Sheffield, 2013).

41 John D. Gilleard and Law Chi-keung Tarcisius, 'Improving the delivery of patient services: alternative workplace strategies in action', *Facilities,* 21, no. 1/2 (2003), 20–7, https://doi.org/10.1108/02632770310460513.

42 Millie A. Harrison, William R. Smith, Mackenzie R. Greenwell and Keri K. Stephens, 'Frontline employees in the health clinic: impression management multiplexing when performing in-the-round', *Communication Monographs,* 85, no. 3 (2018), 309–30, https://doi.org/10.1080/03637751.2018.1429638.

43 Rosica Pachilova and Kerstin Sailer, 'Providing care quality by design: a new measure to assess hospital ward layouts', *The Journal of Architecture,* 25, no. 2 (2020), 186–202, https://doi.org/10.1080/13602365.2020.1733802.

44 Full details can be found in Rosica Pachilova, 'Exploring quality of care in hospital wards: The effect of spatial layout, staff work activities and communication patterns' (PhD, UCL, 2020). https://discovery.ucl.ac.uk/id/eprint/10093866/.

45 Healthcare quality was defined by the Care Quality Commission, which is an independent regulator of all health and social care services in England. It conducts inspections of hospitals and rates them on a four-point scale: outstanding; good; requires improvement; and inadequate. The rating is based on a number of data sources including evidence and information collected throughout their work, feedback and inspections carried out by experts. What the regulatory body monitors as care quality is: safety; team effectiveness; staff care; treating patients with care; dignity and respect; responsiveness to patient needs; leadership; and management of the hospital.

46 Roger Ulrich, Craig Zimring, Xuemei Zhu, Jennifer Dubose, Hyun-Bo Seo, Young-Seon Choi, Xiaobo Quan and Anjali Joseph, 'A review of the research literature on evidence-based healthcare design', *HERD,* 1, 3 (2008), 61–125.

47 Visual connectivity is a local measure which illustrates what one can see within 360 degrees from a single vantage point. It counts all points that are visible from the point of interest as connectivity value and is therefore equivalent to the size of the local viewshed area. This is done for every point on the plan. Points with high visual connectivity values are coloured in red and the smaller the value becomes, the cooler the colour gets.

48 Upali Nanda, Pamela Redden and Richard Ruckstadel, 'Care coordination in oncology: lessons from the field' (paper presented at the Healthcare Design Conference, 2015).

49 T. Manser, 'Teamwork and patient safety in dynamic domains of healthcare: a review of the literature', *Acta Anaesthesiologica Scandinavica*, 53, no. 2 (February 2009): 143–51.

50 Upali Nanda and Deborah Wingler, 'Practice-based research methods and tools: introducing the design diagnostic', *HERD,* 13, no. 4 (2020): 11–26. https://doi.org/10.1177/1937586720945176.

51 Babak Soleimani, Upali Nanda and Sally Augustine, 'Brain meets building when behavior meets space' (paper presented at the ANFA International Conference, The Academy of Neuroscience for Architecture, 2020).

52 Adeleh Nejati, Ryan Gathman, Upali Nanda, Heath May and Tom Harvey, 'Where research meets design: using parametric modelling to optimize walking distances and enhance workflow' (Center for Advanced Design Research and Evaluation, 2014), https://static1.squarespace.com/static/5595c129e4b02838d1264c98/t/55a6bd34e4b07971267c8492/1436990772013/WHDPaperCADRETechnicalReport-141111.pdf.

53 Julie Zook, Kate Renner and Upali Nanda, 'ICU as informational interface: a model for data-driven ICU design' (paper presented at the 12th International Space Syntax Symposium, Beijing, China, 2019).

54 Nanda, Pati and Nejati, 'Field research and parametric analysis in a medical-surgical unit', 11–26.

References

Allen, Davina, 'Re-reading nursing and re-writing practice: towards an empirically based reformulation of the nursing mandate', *Nursing Inquiry,* 11, no. 4 (2004), 271–83, https://doi.org/10.1111/j.1440-1800.2004.00234.x.

Backhouse, Alan, and Peter Drew, 'The design implications of social interaction in a workplace setting', *Environment and Planning B: Planning and Design*, 19 (1992), 573–84.

Becker, Franklin, 'Nursing unit design and communication patterns: what is "real" work?', *HERD,* 1, no. 1 (2007), 58–62, https://doi.org/10.1177/193758670700100115.

Brown, John Seely, and Paul Duguid, 'Organizational learning and communities of practice: toward a unified view of working, learning, and innovation', *Organization Science,* 2, no. 1 (1991), 40–57.

Buerhaus, Peter I., 'Follow-up conversation with Lucian Leape on errors and adverse events in health care', *Nursing Outlook,* 49, no. 2 (2001), 73–7, https://doi.org/10.1067/mno.2001.114404.

Carthey, Jane, 'Reinterpreting the hospital corridor: "wasted space" or essential for quality multidisciplinary clinical care?', *HERD,* 2, no. 1 (2008), 17–29 https://doi.org/10.1177/193758670800200103.

Choudhary, Ruchi, Sonit Bafna, Yeonsook Heo, Ann L. Hendrich and Marilyn Chow, 'A predictive model for computing the influence of space layouts on nurses' movement in hospital units', *Journal of Building Performance Simulation,* 3, no. 3 (2010), 171–84, https://doi.org/10.1080/19401490903174280.

Christensen, Caryn, and James R. Larson, 'Collaborative Medical Decision Making', *Medical Decision Making,* 13, no. 4 (1993), 339–46, https://doi.org/10.1177/0272989x9301300410.

Davies, Celia, 'Getting health professionals to work together: There's more to collaboration than simply working side by side', *BMJ,* 320, no. 7241 (2000), 1021–2, https://doi.org/10.1136/bmj.320.7241.1021.

Donchin, Yoel, Daniel Gopher, Miriam Olin, Yehuda Badihi, Michal B. Biesky, Charles L. Sprung, Ruven Pizov and Shamay Cotev, 'A look into the nature and causes of human errors in the intensive care unit', *Critical Care Medicine,* 23, no. 2 (1995), 294–300, https://doi.org/10.1097/00003246-199502000-00015.

Drucker, Peter, *Landmarks of Tomorrow* (New York: Harper, 1959).

Durkheim, Emile, *The Division of Labor in Society* (New York: The Free Press, 1893).

Egenes, Karen J., 'History of nursing', in Gayle Roux and Judith Halstead (eds), *Issues and Trends in Nursing: Essential Knowledge for Today and Tomorrow* (Burlington, MA: Jones and Bartlett Publishers, 2009).

Encyclopaedia Britannica, 'History of medicine – Hellenistic and Roman medicine', https://www.britannica.com/science/history-of-medicine/Hellenistic-and-Roman-medicine.

Gilleard, John D., and Law Chi-keung Tarcisius, 'Improving the delivery of patient services: alternative workplace strategies in action', *Facilities,* 21, no. 1/2 (2003), 20–7, https://doi.org/10.1108/02632770310460513.

Goffman, Erving, *The Presentation of Self in Everyday Life (*Harmondsworth: Penguin Books, 1959).

Hall, Kendall K., Demetrios N. Kyriacou, Jonathan A. Handler and James G. Adams, 'Impact of emergency department built environment on timeliness of physician assessment of patients with chest pain', *Environment and Behavior,* 40, no. 2 (2008), 233–48, https://doi.org/10.1177/0013916507311548.

Harrison, Millie A., William R. Smith, Mackenzie R. Greenwell and Keri K. Stephens, 'Frontline employees in the health clinic: impression management multiplexing when performing in-the-round', *Communication Monographs,* 85, no. 3 (2018), 309–30, https://doi.org/10.1080/03637751.2018.1429638.

Henderson, Virginia, 'The nature of nursing', *The American Journal of Nursing,* 64, no. 8 (1964), 62–8.

Hendrich, Ann L., Marilyn P. Chow, Boguslaw A Skierczynski and Zhenqiang Lu, 'A 36-hospital time and motion study: how do medical-surgical nurses spend their time?', *The Permanente Journal,* 12, 3 (2008) 25–34, https://doi.org/10.7812/tpp/08-021.

Iedema, Rick, Debbi Long, Katherine Carroll, Maree Stenglin and Jeffrey Braithwaite, 'Corridor work: how liminal space becomes a resource for handling complexities of multi-disciplinary health care' (paper presented at APROS 11: Asia-Pacific Researchers in Organization Studies 11th International Colloquium, Melbourne, Australia, 2005).

Koutsolampros, Petros, Kerstin Sailer, Tasos Varoudis and Rosie Haslem, 'Dissecting visibility graph analysis: the metrics and their role in understanding workplace human behaviour', in *12th International Space Syntax Symposium* (Beijing: Beijing Jiaotong University, 2019), 1–24 (paper no. 191).

Kranzberg, Melvin, and Michael T. Hannan, 'History of the organization of work', in *Encyclopaedia Britannica,* https://www.britannica.com/topic/history-of-work-organization-648000 (accessed 14 January 2021).

Lewin, Simon, and Scott Reeves, 'Enacting "team" and "teamwork": using Goffman's theory of impression management to illuminate interprofessional practice on hospital wards', *Social Science and Medicine,* 72, no. 10 (2011), 1595–602, https://doi.org/10.1016/j.socscimed.2011.03.037.

Lu, Yi, John Peponis and Craig Zimring, 'Targeted visibility analysis in buildings: correlating targeted visibility analysis with distribution of people and their interactions within an intensive care unit', in Daniel Koch, Lars Marcus and Jesper Steen (eds), *Proceedings of the Seventh International Space Syntax Symposium* (Stockholm: Royal Institute of Technology, 2009), 68.1–68.10.

Lu, Yi, and Craig Zimring, 'Can intensive care staff see their patients? An improved visibility analysis methodology', *Environment and Behavior*, 44, no. 6 (2011), 861–76, https://doi.org/10.1177/0013916511405314.

Manser, T., 'Teamwork and patient safety in dynamic domains of healthcare: a review of the literature', *Acta Anaesthesiologica Scandinavica*, 53, no. 2 (February 2009), 143–51.

Markhede, Henrik, and Daniel Koch, 'Positioning analysis: social structures in configurative modelling' (paper presented at the 6th International Space Syntax Symposium, Istanbul, 2007).
Markus, Thomas A., *Buildings and Power: Freedom and Control in the Origin of Modern Building Types* (London: Routledge, 1993).
Murray, Jenni, *A History of Britain in 21 Women: A Personal Selection* (New York: Simon & Schuster, 2016).
Nanda, Upali, Sipra Pati and Adeleh Nejati, 'Field research and parametric analysis in a medical-surgical unit', *HERD,* 8, no. 4 (2015), 41–57, https://doi.org/10.1177/1937586715577370.
Nanda, Upali, Pamela Redden and Richard Ruckstadel, 'Care coordination in oncology: lessons from the field' (paper presented at the Healthcare Design Conference, 2015).
Nanda, Upali, and Deborah Wingler, 'Practice-based research methods and tools: introducing the design diagnostic', *HERD,* 13, no. 4 (2020), 11–26, https://doi.org/10.1177/1937586720945176.
Nejati, Adeleh, Ryan Gathman, Upali Nanda, Heath May and Tom Harvey, 'Where research meets design: using parametric modelling to optimize walking distances and enhance workflow', Center for Advanced Design Research and Evaluation (2014), https://static1.squarespace.com/static/5595c129e4b02838d1264c98/t/55a6bd34e4b07971267c8492/1436990772013/WHDPaperCADRETechnicalReport-141111.pdf.
Nuffield Provincial Hospitals Trust, *Studies in the Functions and Design of Hospitals* (London: Oxford University Press, 1955)., https://www.nuffieldtrust.org.uk/files/2017-01/functions-and-design-of-hospitals-web-final.pdf
Pachilova, Rosica, 'Exploring quality of care in hospital wards: the effect of spatial layout, staff work activities and communication patterns' (PhD, UCL, 2020), https://discovery.ucl.ac.uk/id/eprint/10093866/.
Pachilova, Rosica, and Kerstin Sailer, 'Evidence-based design: the effect of hospital layouts on the caregiver-patient interfaces' (paper presented at the 2nd European Conference on Design 4 Health, Sheffield, 2013).
Pachilova, Rosica, and Kerstin Sailer, 'Providing care quality by design: a new measure to assess hospital ward layouts', *The Journal of Architecture,* 25, 2 (2020), 186–202, https://doi.org/10.1080/13602365.2020.1733802.
Porter, Roy, 'The patient's view', *Theory and Society,* 14, 2 (1985), 175–98, https://doi.org/10.1007/bf00157532.
Rashid, Mahbub, 'Hospital design and face-to-face interaction among clinicians: a theoretical model', *HERD,* 2, no. 4 (2009), 62–84, https://doi.org/10.1177/193758670900200404.
Smith, Adam, *An Inquiry into the Nature and Causes of the Wealth of Nations* (London: W. Strahan and T. Cadell, 1776).
Soleimani, Babak, Upali Nanda and S. Augustine, 'Brain meets building when behavior meets space' (paper presented at the ANFA International Conference, The Academy of Neuroscience for Architecture, 2020).
Steen, Jesper, 'Spatial and social configurations in offices' (paper presented at the 7th International Space Syntax Symposium, Stockholm, 2009).
Taylor, Frederick W., *The Principles of Scientific Management* (New York: Harper & Brothers, 1911), https://archive.org/details/principlesofscie00taylrich/mode/2up.
Thompson, John D., and Grace Goldin, *The Hospital: A Social and Architectural History* (New Haven CT and London: Yale University Press, 1975).
Ulrich, Roger, Craig Zimring, Xuemei Zhu, Jennifer DuBose, Hyun-Bo Seo, Young-Seon Choi, Xiaobo Quan and Anjali Joseph, 'A review of the research literature on evidence-based healthcare design', *HERD*, 1, 3 (2008), 61–125.
Waber, Ben, Jennifer Magnolfi and Greg Lindsay, 'Workspaces that move people', *Harvard Business Review*, 92, no. 10 (2014), 68–77.
Zook, Julie, Kate Renner and Upali Nanda, 'ICU as informational interface: a model for data-driven ICU design' (paper presented at the 12th International Space Syntax Symposium, Beijing, China, 2019).

Chapter 4 Hallway
Introduction

In this chapter, Julie Zook and Sonit Bafna approach the design of the hospital hallway system with an emphasis on the visitor. They identify the central problem of hospital corridor design as the tension between the complexity of hospital space and the simplicity that visitors seek in navigating it. Visitors try to make sense of two questions as they use corridor space: where they are; and how they are supposed to act.

When designers misunderstand the cognitive dimension of wayfinding, even thoughtful layout concepts can end up creating confusion under use conditions. Confusion in hospital corridors also appears when corridors are designed to give the impression of being hospitality environments or other non-institutional building types. Zook and Bafna argue against this, challenging designers to find ways to convey a constructive institutional character in hospital corridor design.

In his response essay, Carlo Giannasca describes the human centred design process that he uses in developing environmental graphic design for wayfinding in hospitals, emphasising methods that build empathy with end users. Taken together, the chapter and essay provide two sets of guidelines: Zook and Bafna on the perceptual and spatial aspects of corridor system design; and Giannasca on a design process for creative work that centres the user as touchstone.

The visitor and hospital corridor design

Julie Zook and Sonit Bafna

Corridor as place, corridor as linkage

At face value, the only real job of corridors is to enable transport by connecting rooms without disturbing what goes on in them too much. From this point of view, a good corridor system is like a good butler, conveying visitors to locations in such a way as to minimise confusion, fuss and effort, and the best corridor systems are the ones that fall away from awareness, so minute are the demands that they place on attention. This analogy does not hit quite right, though. We know that corridors are something more.

In thinking about what that 'something more' is, we might start by looking at the history of the corridor in institutions. Institutions, by definition, structure social interactions,[1] and institutional corridors can therefore be expected to be about social functions above and beyond transport. Hospitals – like prisons, workhouses and schools – are institutional buildings whose norms lead to consistency in human activity. The architecture of institutions provides the backdrop and conditions that perpetuate institutional norms for behaviour and interaction.[2]

Thomas Markus has described how floorplan layouts perpetuate institutional order by demarcating physical and social boundaries and assigning different types of occupant different rights to space.[3] In Markus's telling, corridors enable institutions to control entire groups of occupants, such as patients, prisoners and students. When patients are isolated in cellular rooms, it is the corridor that enables institutional surveillance and controls of the flow of knowledge, people and things. Yet while corridors, on the one hand, clearly fortify hospital institutional practices, they are on the other hand often the place in hospitals where norms fall apart: a patient is guided to the wrong destination; a nurse corrects a doctor; a visitor cries openly in public.

As an example of the indeterminacy of corridors, we can look to descriptions from Clifford Whittingham Beers' 1910 autobiography, *A Mind that Found Itself*. [4] In it, Beers chronicles his stay in three hospitals for mental illness in the northeast United States, mainly describing how brutal institutional practices counteracted his recovery. When Beers talks about corridors specifically, it is sometimes because he has conscripted them into his attempts to subvert the institution, but more often he portrays corridors as the places where cruel acts are de-robed of their secrecy. Beers describes an attendant who, having knocked a patient to the floor of the corridor, asks Beers, 'Did you see that?', to which Beers replies, 'Yes ... and I'll not forget it'. The attendant scoffs at Beers' capacity to act on what he has seen, though Beers' witness is a form of solidarity.

In recent decades, and with exception for pandemic conditions, hospitals in the United States have opened up to visitors. Restricted visiting hours to inpatient wards have given way to policies and spaces that encourage the continuous presence of patient companions. So-called 'family zones' in patient rooms aim to dedicate a place for the visitor, typically a small area along the window wall that is surplus to and outside of the patient care zone. However, and in spite of the shift towards patient and family-centred care, patients and visitors in hospitals are in a confusing position. They have some status or rights to space, but not such that they are emancipated to act freely on their environment, which, in the end, is still a specific kind of institution. This self-contradictory position would seem to prime them to be on the lookout for cues regarding where they are permitted to be and what they are permitted to do. The family zone islands the visitor at a terminus of what is often a complex and confusing sequence of spaces from the public entry of the hospital to the patient room. This sequence is mostly made up of the public corridor system of hospitals and it teems with problems of ambiguity.

The public corridor system of a hospital includes the hallways and the various seating areas and lobbies that open to them. As a spatial system, corridors ought to work to connect the functional units of a hospital, be intelligible for use and imprint the visitor with the image of the institution. In practice, however, hospital designers struggle to provide basic support for navigation, let alone a heartening experience of the relationship between the hospital and the individuals who enter it. Corridors are fundamentally in-between spaces that emanate mixed signals about what activities are meant to happen in them. When corridors are confusing, it is not just that the visitor is incapacitated in matters of wayfinding and orientation, but that the visitor is confused about how to *be*. When entering an institutional setting, a person usually gets pressed into a role – patient, visitor, applicant for a driving licence – and they are supposed to modulate their behaviour accordingly. (We are here following Goffman's description of the dramaturgical dimension of social life.[5]) Hospital corridors are often the kind of spaces where there is a gap between a person's role in an institution and how the architectural environment signals at them.

We need look no further than crowd-sourced reviews of hospitals on a popular consumer review website[6] to get a sense of the discomfort that hospital corridor systems provoke in a variety of hospitals, these in the southeast United States.

Some descriptions focus on knowing where one is:

> I love the suited greeters spread throughout the hospital who greet you with a friendly 'good morning' or 'good afternoon' and offer to help you find your destination. Such a great touch. Like having a concierge around every corner.
>
> Ingrid, K., Stoneridge, Virginia

> they have a lot of people directing patients around so you do not get lost (it's very nice).
>
> Kristine C., Annapolis, Maryland

> I am also not a fan of trying to find my way around such a huge place with A LOT of people who aren't paying attention.
>
> Noelle S., Marietta, Georgia

> Here to visit a friend & family … all employees there very helpful it was a big hospital I don't know where to go and they Took me all the way to my friends room
>
> Amar P., McDonough, Georgia

But other descriptions allude to a more fundamental confusion about the nature of the hospital corridor system and how one is meant to think, feel and act:

> the facilities, though new, are just as cramped and nonsensical as the old buildings. [T]he waiting rooms are in the hallways – there's absolutely no privacy.
>
> Licorice G., Arlington, Virginia

> It is a very nice and clean hospital. The main lobby is beautiful … They have several exhibits such as the aviary exhibit inside with live birds and a garden/pond with fishes.
>
> Phong, T., Smyrna, Georgia

> So I had the safety officer question me about taking a selfie
>
> LeAnn B., Philadelphia, Pennsylvania

> There were people here who looked like they were looking for a place to hang out, people on laptops having full blown conversations, walking around, tv was blasting, staff flirting with people walking in, nurses picking up their pizza outside (hey they gotta eat), but even worse there was a BBQ going on outside in the street serving workers (this is not a joke …), it was a madhouse. Half the crowd looked like they were just hanging out and the rest looked like they actually had a medical emergency. I never saw something like this in my life.
>
> Eric M., Elizabeth, New Jersey

> The reject case from any Zombie movie mill about outside and inside.
>
> Damien B., Atlanta, Georgia

These visitors are describing incongruities as they looked for cues about how to feel and act: waiting rooms too much in the stream of foot traffic, place imageability together with reflexive limits on photography and party activities simultaneous and collocated with medical emergencies.[7]

The visitor comments focus on two quite different things: how to find places and how to feel, think and act. We will take up the issue of corridor layout and wayfinding in the following section and the issue of how the look and feel of corridors inform the visitor experience at the end of this chapter.

Where to go: the layout of corridor systems

The inherent conflict in designing hospital corridor systems is between the physical and organisational complexity of hospitals and the visitor's need for navigable, intelligible space. No one aims to design confusing buildings, but, also, no one really knows how to ensure that perceiving, moving visitors in a hospital will be able to understand where they are and where they are going. Intelligible corridor design would seem to depend on tacit qualities, rather than the explicit ones that are captured in hospital design guidelines on corridor attributes such as minimum widths and maximum egress distances.

Corridor systems function at a cognitive level, as systems to learn, call to mind and navigate. If we are to understand how to design navigable corridors, there is no getting around the need to understand some things about human cognitive abilities. But when we turn to the research literature on spatial cognition, we find insights that are generally unfamiliar to architects, and these lead us to advocate a particular set of design guidelines for hospital corridor systems.

The elusive map in the head

Our cognitive ability to learn, store and then retrieve environmental knowledge seems to require some kind of a representation of environment in the mind. And the existence of 'cognitive maps' is exactly what early psychologists discovered when investigating spatial problem solving in rats.[8] Since then, the character of the cognitive map has been in question: especially, how knowledge for cognitive maps is acquired and what form it is stored in.

Conventionally, this knowledge is conceived as taking two very distinct formats.[9] One format consists of sequences of instructions that allow us to go from one known location to another; this is known as 'route knowledge'. In the second format, 'survey knowledge', understanding of a learned environment has a configurational and map-like character that includes a sense of the geometrical relationships between different features of the environment.[10] The distinction seems natural enough to be obvious because it conforms to everyday experiences of solving navigational problems. We have all had the experience of following step-by-step instructions when looking for a specific place and also of bringing to the mind some map-like image of a place that we are navigating. Survey knowledge is held to be superior to route knowledge, because its map-likeness allows us a greater range of self-directed actions, such as planning alternatives routes, correcting navigational errors and keeping ourselves orientated with respect to the entire geography of an area.

Calling on survey knowledge, as an experience, can feel like referring to a visual image of the layout, and it may be partly for this reason that survey knowledge is often conceived literally: as a map in the head with actual map- or image-like qualities. While there has long been indication that the structure of knowledge in our head is probably not all that map-like, researchers still occasionally slip back into the analogy: 'Survey-level knowledge is often described as the ability to discern elements in the environment "from a bird's-eye view"'.[11]

The idealised 'map in the head' has shaped researchers' conceptions of the way that layout knowledge is acquired. In this account – which, again, seems natural enough – acquisition of knowledge begins with learning about specific landmarks or locations, which are then assembled to create route knowledge. Then, as in-between areas become filled in, the disparate knowledge of routes is integrated into a single map that acts as a foundation for survey knowledge.[12] The end result of this process is conceived as a map that is densely filled in with all kinds of detail – not only geometrical relations between elements, but also imagistic features – until it is as complete as possible, limited mainly by the brain's memory storage capacities. The key learning operation characterising this development is *integration*, the mechanism by which disparate routes and landmark memories are assembled into a single, coherent map.

This model of knowledge acquisition has been questioned lately, with some researchers positing that survey knowledge begins to emerge quite early in our acquaintance with a new environment, in combination with route and landmark knowledge, and that it is gradually enriched as routes and landmarks are added and their relationships clarified. Nevertheless, this slightly different approach tends to lead to the same ends as prior approaches. Both conceptions distinguish route and survey knowledge and both take the quality of survey knowledge as important to an individual's ability to navigate. Recent research shows the hold that these two fundamental ideas still have on researchers' conceptions of the knowledge of layout.[13]

Architectural wayfinding

The idea of a 'map in the head as an image' has been translated quite directly into design guidelines on corridor layouts for complex buildings, such as hospitals. For such guidelines, the central – and mistaken – thesis is that *good layouts are imageable layouts*, with 'good' in this case meaning that they have forms that are easy to learn, memorise and recall and 'imageable' meaning that they have a strong visual form in plan view. Consider the following recommendations from a standard-setting text on architectural wayfinding and corridor design:[14]

1. Simplicity, characterised by the goodness of form (or *gestalt*) of the figure of the floorplan, especially the form of the corridor system.
2. Clear articulation of the individual corridors through prominent nodes and junctions, which is, again, argued on the basis of easily recognisable graphic form.
3. Regular grid organisation, as long as the layouts also meet the two criteria above.
4. Symmetry and repetition, both of which can be understood as elaborations of the desired gestalt qualities.
5. Close match between volumetric organisation of the building and shape of the corridor system in plan to support users in making inferences about the shape of the plan when navigating it from inside.
6. Shallow hierarchy within the corridor system, which is slightly surprising, but it is argued on the grounds that hierarchy can increase the visual complexity of the figure, and thus make it more difficult to call it to mind.

Even the authors of these suggestions end up recognising that following them does not necessarily lead to the desired results. The text above ends with an instance of a building that embodies the desired characteristics, but, as the authors acknowledge: 'The symmetrical layout of Saint Mary's Hospital in Milwaukee must have disoriented more than an occasional visitor.'[15]

Empirical studies of wayfinding are awash with results indicating that people are just not that good at mentally constructing and using image-like maps. In a study of layout knowledge among students at a medical school, there was little similarity across the maps of a building floor drawn from memory by third-year students. Idiosyncrasy persisted where one might expect convergence and consistency after years of using a space. When compared with first-year students, the third-year students were able to label more places on their maps, but they also made four times as many errors.[16] If exposure led to survey knowledge, which in turn led to a map in the head, maps drawn from memory would neither vary so widely nor become less accurate over repeated exposure. Even when experiment participants are provided with map images for learning layouts, they do not necessarily perform better than participants without maps.[17] When faced with complex three-dimensional environments, they favour route-learning strategies over map-learning ones.[18] Wayfinding design strategies based on creating a readily imageable plan view of the corridor system do not seem to work that well. If an imageable plan does little to aid wayfinding, we are left to ask what does?

Cognitive maps

A development in the neurology of cognitive maps gives us insight into another way of thinking about the problem. This development is the discovery – due primarily to the work of John O'Keefe and colleagues – of the mechanism by which a mapping of the environment occurs in the brain, specifically in the hippocampus.[19]

What O'Keefe and others found was that when an animal[20] finds itself in a recognised location in an environment, the event is signalled by the firing of specific cells in the hippocampus. Learning an environment involves a process of training specific cells to fire in the context of a specific location. The most common of these calls are called 'place cells'. The place cells recognise their location by responding to a particular configuration of a discrete set of cues discerned in the environment and storing information that codes for a vector originating at the centroid of the cues and ending at the actual location of organism. There is much intricate detail about hippocampal activity that this work has uncovered, and much remains to be understood, but this brief description is enough for us to draw two points of relevance.

First, this mode of coding locations frees the animal from a strictly egocentric perspective, at least within limited regions of a layout. So long as the set of cues describing an environment remains consistent, changes of positions and orientations are simply registered as changes in the length and direction of the vector, allowing the individual to keep orientated even as their position changes with respect to the cues. The implication is that the individual can develop knowledge of environmental layout based on a frame of reference centred on the environment itself.[21] (It is important to bear in mind, however, that O'Keefe and others' work has been conducted almost exclusively on animals in settings that are spatially constrained to a specific set of visual cues, often mazes or laboratory rooms within which mazes are placed. These studies have not yet shown a how a complex layout like a plan of a hospital can be entirely captured in a single hippocampal map.[22])

Second, the hippocampal model of spatial learning brings home an unexpected but very significant point: that the hippocampal map is not properly a speaking a map at all, but is instead a *record* of the features that are salient to the animal learning it. Instead of thinking of the hippocampal map as encoding the geometry of the layout in the same way that geographic information system (GIS) maps are loaded into navigational systems, we would do better to think of hippocampal maps as being like a collection of sensors. Learning an environment, then, consists of training dedicated and specific sets of sensors to activate when in specific locations in a given environment.[23] In this map-as-sensor model, all that is needed for learning a layout is the training of sensors, a memory for the set of cues that define a location, and a memory of cues that define adjoining locations. Having developed these, a navigating animal can know where it is once placed in the environment and can predict locations adjoining it. This information should be sufficient to navigate even a complex layout.

There is no need for an individual to store a comprehensive map and develop complex procedures for translating information from the map into instructions for navigation. A person with a map-as-sensor knowledge of the environment will behave exactly like the test subjects of the navigational experiments we encountered above; they can find their way around in environments with complex layouts without necessarily possessing the ability to describe or draw the layout, or even to point accurately to unseen locations.

It may be objected that we nevertheless bring map-like images to mind for specific kinds of spatial or navigational problem. However, this happens only when we address specific problems *whose solutions require information not available in our visible surroundings* – for instance, deciding whether one route is longer than another. We do produce map-like images in our minds in these situations, but these maps need only be quite diagrammatic. Research on the psychology of spatial memory often affirms that image-like maps of layouts that people bring to mind are not only diagrammatic but are invariably distorted, simplified, lacking in detail and fragmented.[24] What is more, the distortions have a predictable character: crooked lines are straightened, angles near 90 degrees are rounded to make right-angled corners and minor mismatches are ignored. The schematic character of these maps is often taken as evidence of partial or mistaken knowledge, but the deformations are more feature than bug. The task of these maps is not to depict the environment, but to support reasoning for specific problems. They are, in effect, mental models.[25]

The main insight from this discussion is that a person navigating a space confronts two kinds of problem that require distinct capabilities. The first kind we solve when situated in a place without visualising in advance the shape of a route that we intend to take. The cognitive system that makes this possible – the centrepiece of which is the hippocampal cognitive map – is always active and can run even when we are distracted or not consciously attending to the navigational task.[26] The second kind of problem concerns strategies for environments from which we are removed or that we are otherwise actively trying to learn. When faced with these kinds of problem, we rely on a set of general spatial problem-solving abilities to create highly schematic map-like images to aid in solving navigational problems.[27] This construction of map-like mental models of the environment is cognitively demanding and needs dedicated attentional resources.

Much of the current guidance for architectural wayfinding mixes the two kinds of cognitive task: the background learning that takes place via hippocampal maps; and the active learning that takes place when we try to construct mental maps of places. The result is recommendations that, as reasonable as they are at face value, often miss their mark.

Design and navigational problems

People familiar with a building mostly navigate without calling to mind mental maps of their environments. Visitors and short-term occupants, on the other hand, abound in hospitals, and they might more often need to construct mental maps as they try to plan routes or maintain orientation. Typically, a partial map is all visitors need; they are not navigating whole hospitals, but only trying to get to a specific destination. The remainder of this section focuses on the kinds of problems faced by visitors and other users new to a space.

Visitors resort to visualising mental maps for two main reasons: to find quick solutions to navigational problems and to aid gradual learning over repeat visits. A key requirement of the designed environment in both cases is to provide cues that support visitors in constructing effective mental models of specific wayfinding tasks.

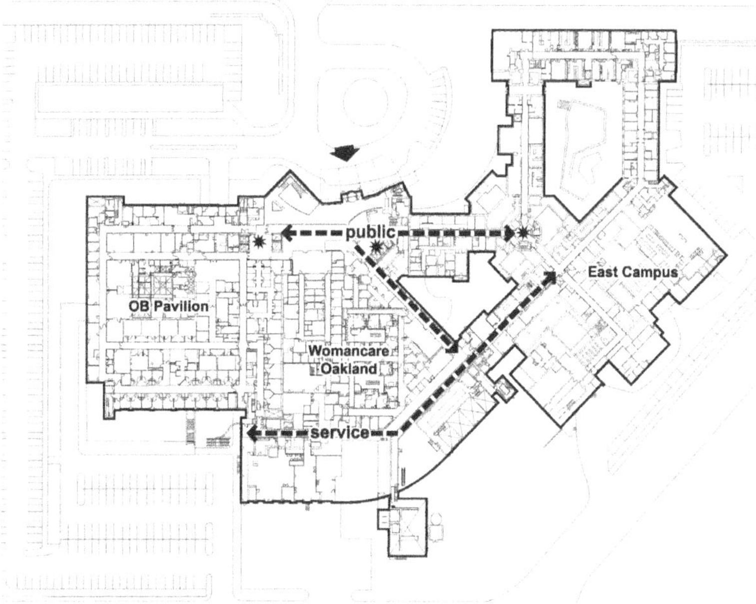

4.1 A well-designed hospital with a challenging corridor system. Tsoi Kobus, used with permission, 2021.

Even good designers who are focused on navigational simplicity can create conditions that hinder wayfinding. In the first plan (see Figure 4.1), the public circulation focuses on the main entrance lobby (marked by a large arrow) and branches out from there radially, leading to different sub-areas. As a scheme, the organisation of the hospital is exceptionally easy to read in plan, with marked shifts in the orientation of corridors and rooms demarcating sub-areas that correspond to distinct programmatic units. The break in the geometry also calls out the entrance and disrupts the rigidity of the otherwise orthogonal blocks. The organising grids of the three main areas are reflected in the pattern of their major internal corridors. The design literally makes the entire hospital visitor-centred in the sense of minimising the distances to different sub-areas of the hospital from the public entrance. The circulation structure also has a good gestalt, in the sense that the overall shape of the major corridors is an imageable geometric form. The diagrammatic redrawing of the plan makes these points visually explicit (see Figure 4.2).

However, the diagrammatic redrawing also illustrates a characteristic feature that increases wayfinding difficulty. The use of triangular blocks results in some corridors that are turned 45 degrees with respect to the others. While this creates memorable form as the

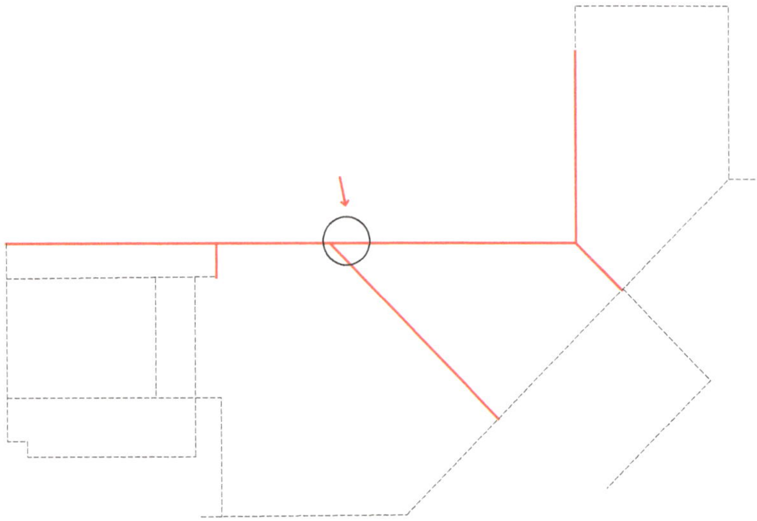

4.2 Diagrammatic redrawing of hospital corridor plan.

image of the plan, on the ground it will likely be highly disorientating because corridors with turns of about 45 degrees tend to create navigational problems.[28] In both laboratory[29] and urban-based[30] experiments, path segments at or around 45 degrees from a reference path resulted in poor performance on navigation tasks. People use perceptual cues from the immediate environment – especially those related to an overall directional framework – to make inferences about orientation. For orientation in new environments, 45-degree lines of movement are likely to increase the chance of making errors.

Graphic strategies for a good plan-view gestalt too often correspond to *in situ* spatial conditions that confuse and undermine navigation, especially for visitors unfamiliar with a place. Corridor designs that work against basic navigational tendencies often end up loaded with compensatory features and practices: colour-coded hospital zones, special maps (app-based or on paper), lines on the floor leading to various departments, complex and elaborate systems of signage and dedicated greeters or concierge to direct building users. These strategies herald failures in spatial design. Below, we discuss how approaches to the design of corridor layouts might better aid visitors in their quest to both solve immediate navigational tasks and learn a layout for future use.

Layouts that lend themselves to being learned

A layout that lends itself to mental modelling is one that lets you distil a framework of key corridors from among the large number of hallways that constitute a complex building, like a hospital. Some guidelines to this end follow:

1. A good general strategy is to design layouts with an armature of corridors that have a hierarchy that registers during use and to design this armature to have good reach, in the sense of providing access to various parts of the layout.

This could mean having few major corridors that reach more or less straight across the extent of a building, connecting its main areas and branching off into minor corridors. Working from a robustly navigable spatial core, detailed design decisions can reinforce the hierarchy by marking the transitions to the secondary corridors through changes in size or visual character.

There are also several corridor conditions to avoid:

2. Corridors that meet each other at angles near 45 degrees are disorientating and should be avoided, although occasional small turns in corridors (less than 15 degrees)[31] can provide flexibility or ease the severity of a plan without compromising its navigability. (These small deflections seem to be 'rounded' to continuous straight lines in the mind.)
3. Corridors that do not continue through, but are slightly offset, creating T-junctions, increase the complexity and navigational difficulty of a layout.
4. Major corridors that create loops with legs that cannot be distinguished because they lack perceptual and cognitive hierarchy and are therefore disorientating.

The fundamental recommendations, towards spatial and perceptual order, become hard to achieve because complex corridors systems have intrinsic hierarchies based on patterns of connection that are not necessarily perceptible. When designers fail to recognise these underlying spatial patterns, physical design or programming along corridors can be mistmatched with patterns of actual use.

Approaches from space syntax enable insights about hierarchies in corridor systems by representing and analysing the layout of corridors as a network of nodes (corridors) and links (intersections). Treating corridors as elements of a graph allows us to uncover latent hierarchies and differences in terms of their 'syntactic' properties.

A very early finding in space syntax studies was that the integration values for hospital corridors[32] were a clear predictor of the frequency of use in open-ended exploratory navigation by visitors unfamiliar with the layout.[33] The study revealed common disconnects between design intent and design performance. While the front-of-house corridor was intended to act as a spine and reference for navigating subjects, it was the more integrated corridor at the back of the plan that actually did so. The integrated portions of the corridor system appeared to anchor cognitive maps, as participants returned more frequently to them while they aimed to get to know the layout (during exploratory search). Another study of a large public hospital occupying an entire urban block confirmed these findings.[34] In addition, the researchers also found that the visitors unfamiliar with the hospital, tended to learn very quickly – within about 15 minutes – to move to the most integrated areas while solving wayfinding tasks.

Typically, hospital layouts are structured in such a way that lobbies and public areas end up with high integration values, and in this way the hospital type can form a basis for roughly aligning well-integrated spaces with the public corridor programme. However, ensuring hierarchy within the corridor system is another task. One can run a syntax analysis of a floorplan, but, in cases where that is not feasible one can follow the guidelines below. These add details to strategies raised above and are aimed at capturing basic layout strategies for a corridor system that gains navigability from hierarchies:

5. The layout should be organised around a core of a few, relatively straight-running primary corridors that are directly connected to each other, and these primary corridors should span the layout as much as possible. A long corridor that is weakly linked will not function well as a primary corridor and will probably lead to wayfinding problems.
   Buildings can also maintain a simple set of primary corridors by 'offloading' some of the circulatory work into distinct and bounded areas, such as hospital departments, that connect strategically to the primary corridor systems and have their own internal circulatory logic.

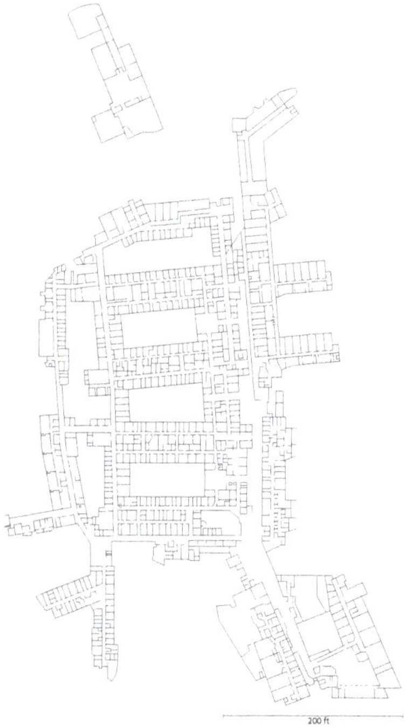

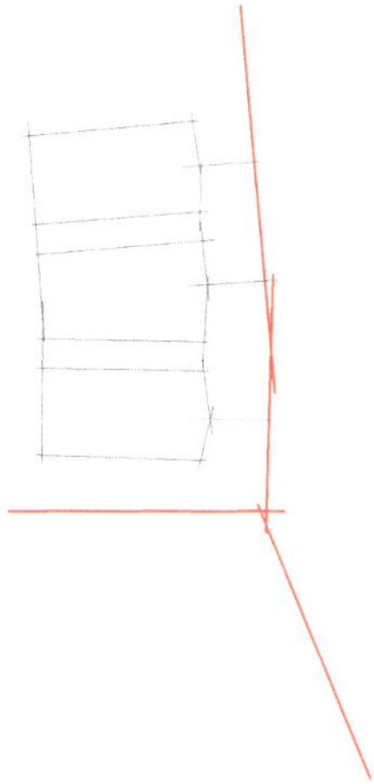

4.3 The plan and corridor system at Rikshospitalet (right). Drawn by Victor Carrillo and Daniel Rios, 2021.

4.4 Diagrammatic redrawing of Rikshospitalet corridor plan (left).

The floorplan layout of the Rikshospitalet in Oslo provides an example of several of these guidelines, including a corridor hierarchy that is perceptible; a long corridor that spans the layout and connects its parts; small deflections that break up the longest corridor without driving up plan complexity and linkages to departments that act as districts unto themselves (see Figures 4.3 and 4.4).

The key insight presented here is that designing to support navigation in complex buildings should proceed from understanding the actual kinds of problem that people are trying to solve, as well as the kinds of cognitive capacity that they usually bring to them. Building visitors can navigate without first – or ever – constructing extensive, rich, unitary mental maps of entire layouts in their heads. The guidelines above are aimed at supporting design based on these premises.

In addition to their function in constituting navigable systems of spaces, an equally significant impact of hospital corridor systems comes through the way that they look and feel. It is through their look and feel, aided to some extent by their organisation, that corridors help to construct and maintain the hospital as an institution, and, moreover, to modulate the subjectivity of individual visitors and staff.

How to be: the look and feel of corridor systems

The hospital as a building type is an institution characterised by somewhat coercive norms for interaction and behaviour.[35] This condition seems linked to a belief that the architectural inscription of institutionality in contemporary environments such as hospitals, leads to deleterious effects.[36] It is perhaps in reaction to the negative perception of institutional norms that some typical approaches to shaping hospital corridor interiors seem aimed at suppressing the identity of the hospital as an institution, or at least toning it down to suggest a more relaxed and flexible kind of

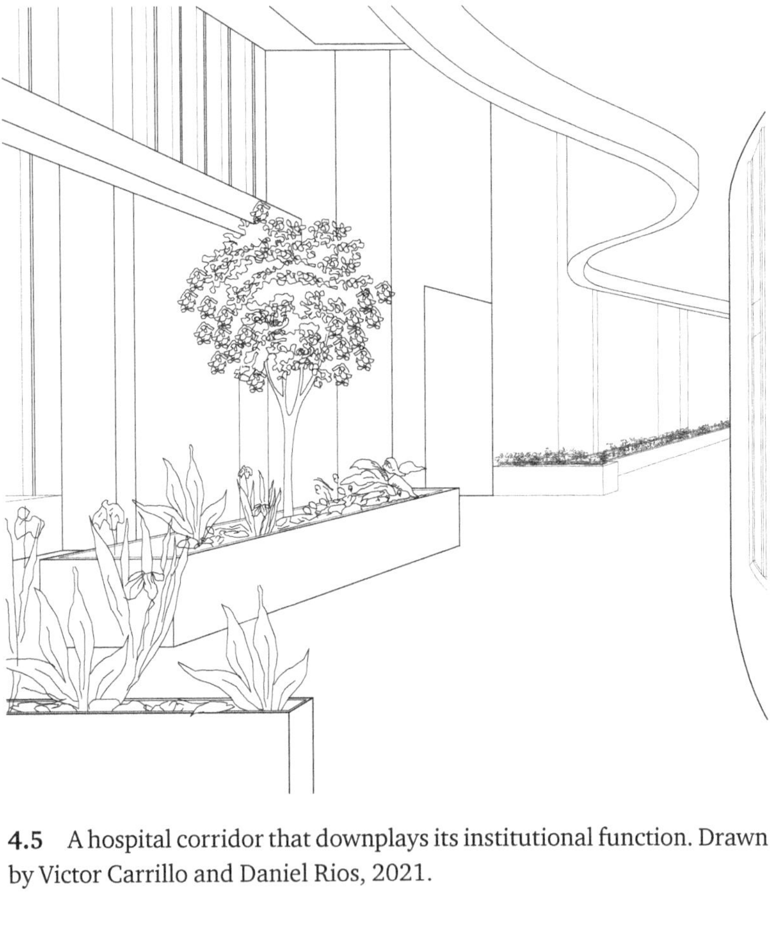

4.5 A hospital corridor that downplays its institutional function. Drawn by Victor Carrillo and Daniel Rios, 2021.

institution. For example, the hospital corridor above (see Figure 4.5 adapted from a photograph) passes through terraced planters and is framed by curving walls and areas enriched with seating, while features of the wall and ceiling are elaborated in ways that break up orthogonality. But such approaches seem ineffectual against the numbing sense that coercive environments can create.

The problem is that designers cannot simply bolt a hospitality-style corridor onto departments designed in a functionalist mode and hope that the intimations of hotel or corporate lounges in public areas will dispel a negative sense of institutional character. The 'tale of two aesthetics' that this promotes reduces the perceived coherence of the hospital as an institution. On one hand, it heightens the effect of the impersonal structuring of the department areas, with their highly partitioned spaces, rigidly classified activities and generic selection of furnishings and finishes. On the other, it downplays the presentation of the hospital in the public areas, for example by offering the image of a corporate lobby or hotel instead of that of a hospital. Denying the hospital a distinctive visual character in its own right acknowledges, in a backhanded way, distrust in the hospital as an institution.

It is, in other words, futile to malign or suppress institutionality as such, because hospitals are inevitably institutions. A hospital's institutionality is among its assets because the consistent nature of institutions underlies the social trust that a hospital will reliably purvey medical examination and treatment. The source of the perceived banality and oppressiveness in so many hospitals may be less their institutionality in general and more the appearance of a specific form of institutionality that comes across as impersonal and unempathetic. When regulatory social norms are perceived as being governed by strong classificatory system, the system will appear to dominate individual volition, such as the volition of patients and their caregivers.[37]

Hospital corridor design can counter the atmosphere or feel of oppressive institutionality that emerges in hospitals. The public corridor system of a hospital is the space that most closely approximates universal inclusion and mixing of role types. Hospital corridor systems therefore have the potential to act as liminal behaviour settings,[38] where rules and roles are not given as a natural outcome of an impersonal institution, but, rather, are available as negotiable and malleable through individual interaction. The effect of this can be to create an institutional setting in which genuine human exchange is possible. Producing a positive architectural sense of institutionality is both a matter of adjusting norms and behaviour and of establishing the right look and feel in the spaces.

Institutionality is not simply a matter of social practice but also of projected image. The image matters because institutions need to exist as a coherent collective thought – an image – in the minds of their members in order to maintain themselves.[39] Projection of a consistent image can be a means not only of expressing the hospital's instrumental values (standardly, cleanliness, efficiency and reliability) but also of conveying the social values of individual volition and personal negotiation over systemic control.

Consider the Gregorio Marañón Maternity and Paediatric Hospital in Madrid, designed by the office of Rafael Moneo and executed between 1997 and 2003 – a building recognised for its image as much for its functionality.[40] The overall conceptual form of the building is organised as four aligned major courtyards that organise the wards, staff spaces and a grid of corridors (see Figure 4.6). The result is a floorplan composed entirely of rectilinear spaces, with no curves, rotations or even overlapped rectangles appearing anywhere. The exterior is characterised by horizontal metal panels, the protruding seams of which extend across the fenestration and regulate window size and location. A multi-storey glazed volume signals the public entrance.

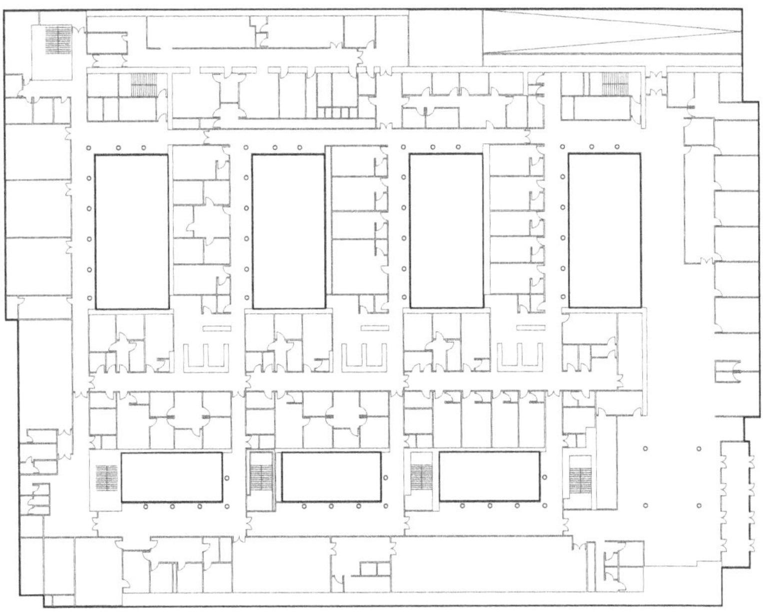

4.6 A floorplan of the Gregorio Marañón Maternity and Paediatric Hospital in Madrid. Drawn by Victor Carrillo and Daniel Rios, 2021.

At first glance, these decisions have the effect of presenting the hospital as an institution unambiguously organised around operational demands and basic environmental requirements, such as adequate daylight and visual exposure to natural elements. Features such as the sense of purposefulness in the facades and the perceptible fit-to-function nature of the circulatory system work together to project an institutional character that emphasises efficiency, no-nonsense functioning and rationality. At a basic perceptual level, the interior of the hospital expresses well-understood and uncontroversial values associated with modern medical practice (i.e., hygiene and efficiency).[41]

What makes this hospital a compelling example for us is the way that it manages to convey a sense of the personal in how the design appears. First, there is an unusual level of formal consistency throughout all parts of the building. The visual character of the hospital is similar in its offices, corridors, treatment rooms and patient rooms. These spaces, which accommodate different roles and activities, share an aesthetic and level of finish. There is no divided aesthetic, with the implication of a foundation of solidarity among the building's many occupant roles.

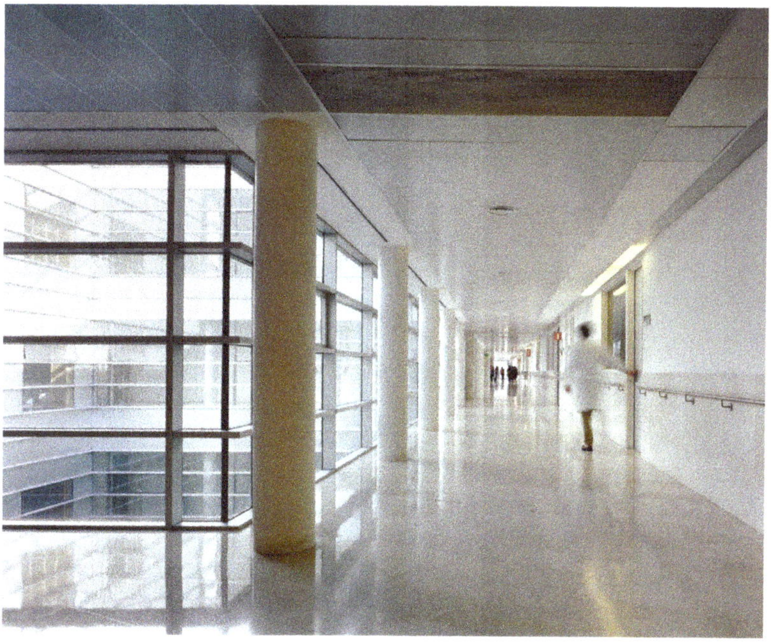

4.7 A corridor at the Gregorio Marañón Maternity and Paediatric Hospital. Copyright Michael Moran/OTTO.

Second, there is a constant effort made to acknowledge basic human perceptual faculties and tendencies to seek out affordances. The strict geometries of the spaces as they appear in plan are often softened by the handling of their bounding surfaces, particularly the walls and windows. From inside the corridors, for example, the long expanses of glazing are buffered by the structural columns, the depth of which is inscribed in slight changes of the floor and ceiling surfaces, with the window mullions adding additional softness to the expression of planar surfaces (see Figure 4.7). In patient rooms, the exterior wall is broken up by a small interstitial space corresponding to the depth of the wall that opens onto the courtyards, and these openings are lined with pairs of folding louvered doors (see Figure 4.8). Other features – for example, the custom-made, consistent-quality finishes and furniture – obviate the feeling that the building was shaped by generic institutional conventions.

Third, there are signs that consistent care is taken to favour human experience and comfort over considerations of economy and systems efficiency. Corridors are wider and more spacious than required programmatically, so that the entire building appears to have a high ratio of corridor to patient-room area. Even in photographs, it is easy to read the insistence by which the relationship to courtyard is maintained throughout the planning of the building. Many corridors are kept single-loaded, ensuring that they have exposure to light and views offered by the courtyards. This is a typological deviation from the contemporary inpatient ward block, whose forms often express permutations of, but not deviation from, the more efficient double-loaded corridor type.

One interesting way in which the Marañon hospital seems to counter a sense of institutionality is by its display of clear authorial intent. (In the architecture of complex buildings, this is generally the authorial work of a group, not an individual.) Over and above creating desired perceptual qualities, the look and feel of the interior of the hospital conveys the sense that an independent, specific and particular sensibility has prevailed over systemic dictates, though not in an idiosyncratic or whimsical manner. And it does so in at least three distinct ways – consistency of visual character through the functional and public areas; discernible attention to human scale and perceptual tendencies; and explicit signs that human experience is favoured over systemic processes.

There are no formulae for ensuring the right kind of image to counter the sense of impersonal institutionality and neither the Gregorio Marañón Hospital in particular nor Moneo's architecture more generally provide definite exemplars to be followed. Instead, the idea here is in *how*

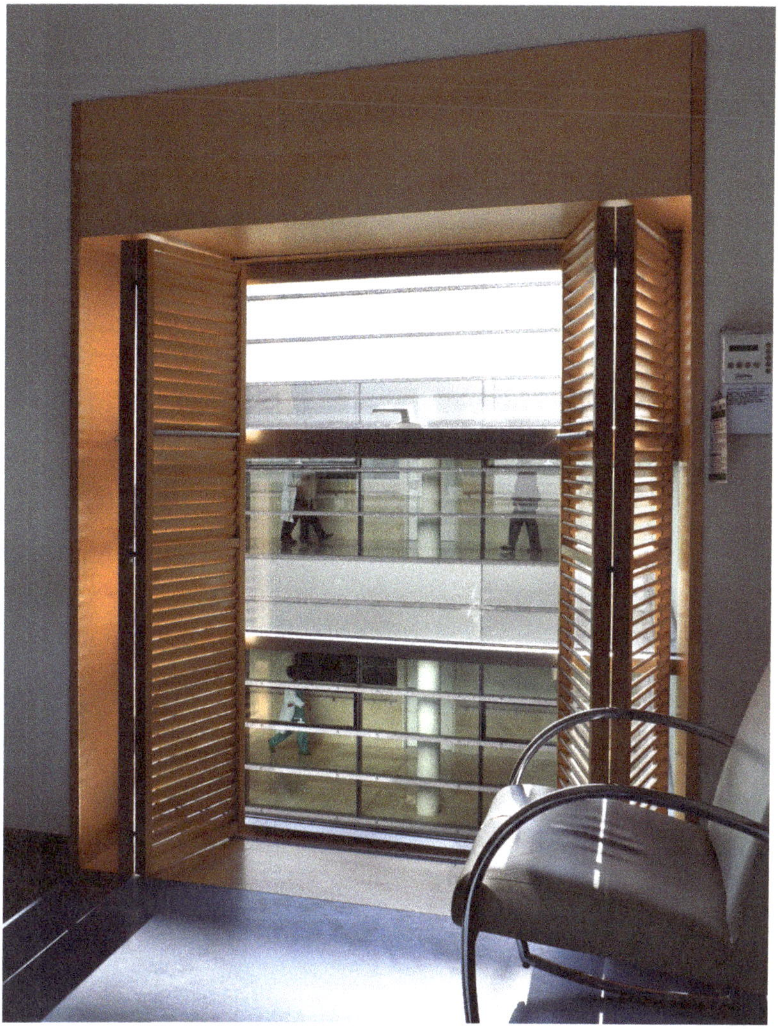

4.8 A patient room at the Gregorio Marañón Maternity and Paediatric Hospital overlooks the corridor. Copyright Michael Moran/OTTO.

the foregrounding of authorial intent is achieved. Our example, we think, clarifies that means to achieve this involve at least:

1. a broad awareness of conventional solutions so that unconventional ones can be proposed;
2. originality in form-making – it need not be visually loud – so that a sense of the personal is consistently discernible in the design; and
3. stylistic consistency to guard against whimsy.

These can be best achieved through disciplined and self-reflective practice.

A parallel distinction between pictorial representations (such as paintings and photographs) and works of art comes into play in evaluating common tendencies in the placement of art in hospital corridors. As work in the philosophy of art has long recognised, an artwork is defined not by classification of a given artefact as such, but by the contemplative engagement with which it is approached and by the relational and institutional contexts in which it is presented. A painting can be a simply pleasing decoration in one context and a work of art in another.[42] In museums, art is often placed with respect to themes, sometimes to advance a pedagogic aim, and museum space affords conditions that are amenable to viewing and reflecting on the work in a fundamentally social way.[43]

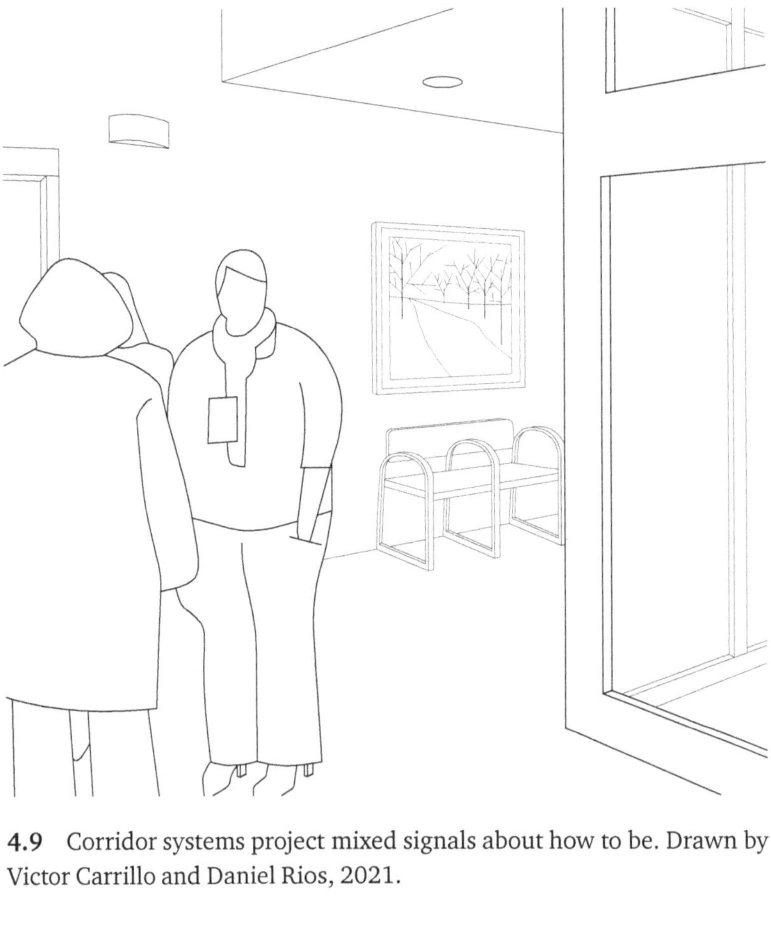

4.9 Corridor systems project mixed signals about how to be. Drawn by Victor Carrillo and Daniel Rios, 2021.

In hospitals, artwork, often in the form of device-based multimedia displays, is sometimes included in treatment areas based on studies indicating that such interventions reduce perceived pain.[44] These studies address situations where the value of art, or art-like artefacts, lies in its ability to distract during experiences of pain (usually physical). In terms of corridors specifically, art is often argued to create a more pleasant ambience, although artwork can act also to fine-tune wayfinding design, as discussed in the essay by Carlo Giannasca that follows.

Problems emerge specifically when hospital artwork is placed without regard for social context. (On walls behind banks of chairs seems a favoured location; Figure 4.9 is drawn from a photo.) In such situations, art is at cross purposes with the social groupings that the hospital space is otherwise laid out to accommodate. When in an exam room, for example, a picture that faces the patient, but not the doctor, undermines the realisation in space of a shared interest – of a provisional joint worldview – between doctor and patient.[45] In such arrangements, hospital art would seem to inadvertently reinforce the divide between socially defined categories.

Corridor systems give architectural form to connections, which is to say that corridors shape the terms of our access to each other. Hospital corridor systems have generative potential, in spite of their history of coercion. They can prompt us away from role-driven self-concepts and behaviours and towards less rigidly arbitrated interactions. They can engage our cognition and imagination. They can create an impression of the specific institution with which we find ourselves engaged. A certain sort of architectural functionalism might evaluate hospital corridor systems purely in terms of minimising travel distances, travel times or percent of total floor area, while a certain squeamishness about institutions might lead a designer to aim to submerge the corridor in decoration and amenity.

In this chapter, we develop two normative statements about corridors. First, corridor systems should answer to the specific capacities of the human cognitive system; and, second, they should be shaped to construct a relation of the individual to the institution. These two questions raised by corridor systems – *where am I? how am I supposed to be?* – correspond to the status of corridors as both collections of networked behaviour settings and as behaviour settings in their own right.

To know where one is, one needs to learn the layout of the system. Where prior design guidelines have assumed the construction of a detailed map-like mental representation, we advocate for an approach that is more attuned to what is presently known about human cognition:

specifically, that we do not need to carry within our head a detailed and complete map-like representation of a layout. Instead, we often learn a layout by creating a cognitive map that is activated only *in situ* and filling in for gaps in knowledge by additional cognitive mapping of partial layouts on an as-needed basis. Layouts, then, are freed from the requirement of being imageable in total and can be shaped to answer the navigational problems of particular kinds of occupant and visitor.

In corridor systems, an institutional morphology of form meets an individual morphology of experience. Corridor system design that suppresses the expression of the hospital as an institution does hospitals and their users a disservice, as though the hospital and its occupants are both somehow in the wrong from the outset. Corridor systems can convey not only the rational and predictable dimensions of hospitals, but can also create visual, spatial and imaginative conditions that add meaning to daily life in institutional settings.

Response Essay: Designing a human -centred hospital wayfinding system

Carlo Giannasca

When we undertake the design of a wayfinding system for healthcare facilities, we adopt a classic human-centred design (HCD) approach to the process. The government in Sydney, Australia has shown foresight that requires design firms to use a clearly prescribed HCD process in the development of public-health infrastructure projects. This requires the design to pass through various stages of rigorous user-testing to ensure that the solutions we develop are validated. We must be far more thorough in our design methodology throughout the whole process to ensure what we create is optimised for success.

When we undertake wayfinding projects in our consultancy, we take our clients through a particular process that is designed to extract as much information as we need to maximise our ability to deliver the best result possible. As such, we follow a five-step HCD process that was originally devised by IDEO.

The first and most critically important step is to start by framing the design challenge. This is done typically by framing the challenge with a question, such as, 'How might we enhance the visitor experience in a hospital through the addition of a comprehensive and comprehendible signage and wayfinding system?' As American inventor Charles F. Kettering once said, 'A problem well stated is a problem half-solved'. Once we have defined the problem, we can start to investigate the user experience and how it can be enhanced.

The second step of the HCD process is to build empathy with the intended audience. The process reinforces that, ultimately, we are designing for people and not just for design's sake. Therefore, we must better understand people and their relationships with their environment, so that we know where that experience can be enhanced or improved. Part of the empathy-building process involves conducting interactive workshops with the various user group representatives and co-creating the brief for the project. This usually includes people from all levels of hospital administration, doctors, nurses, patient and visitor advocacy groups, among others. We have had a lot of success actively involving users in the process because we can directly capture responses and take them on the creative journey from the beginning. To do this effectively, we need to build a profile and create personas of who we are designing for.

To design a truly effective wayfinding system, we must understand:

1. user needs (e.g., finding the main entrance into a building);
2. frustrations (e.g., not knowing how long the wait will be);
3. personal experiences (e.g., keeping children happy in the waiting room);
4. particular characteristics (e.g., whether there are any cultural or language barriers);
5. motivations (e.g., key reason for visiting);
6. behaviours (e.g., stress because users are visiting a sick or dying family member);
7. user profile; and
8. user goals.

This information is typically gathered through face-to-face 'in the field' intercept interviews. These 'intercepts' are carried out at the various steps along the user journey. The output is often a chart that captures the data in a digestible and applicable form that can then inform the design process (see Figure 4.10). From the data that we gather, we create a number of different user profiles, which can vary depending on the complexity of the project. Once we have established the various persona types, we begin to map their journey and establish what we want them to think, feel and do along each step of the way. This is shown diagrammatically in Figure 4.10.

We consider what happens before, during and after their visit. By mapping the experience, we can define opportunities and identify where the journey can be enhanced through the use of wayfinding. We further

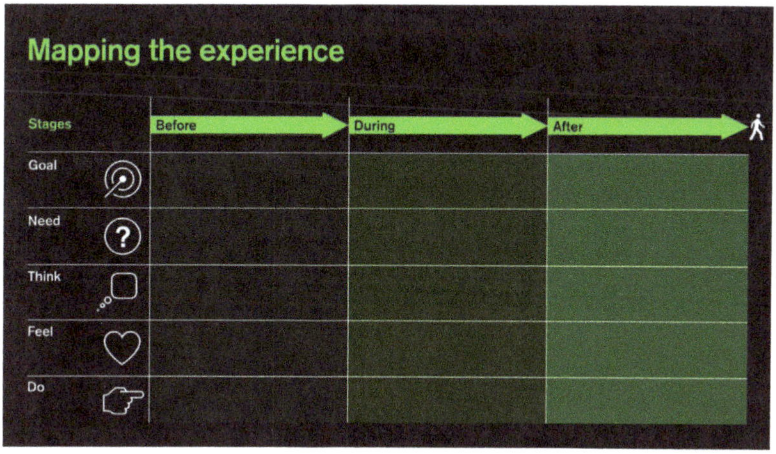

4.10 A chart for building profiles of building users. Image courtesy of Frost Collective.

map for persona types, creating a detailed experience map for every visitor type that we profile. This provides a rich source of data on all that will interact with the building.

In addition to the more conceptual approach to mapping the user journey, we also look at it from a more practical angle. We look at the whole journey sequence from the viewpoint of what signs we specifically need at critical decision points to ensure that the user understands clearly the correct path to take.

The third step in the HCD process is where we start to ideate. For a designer, this is the fun part. This is where we synthesise what we have learned in the empathy-building phase and exercise our creativity. However, designing a great wayfinding system is as much a scientific endeavour as it is an artistic one. We need to appreciate how people understand their environments and what tools we can equip them with to help them on their way.

In his seminal book *The Image of the City*,[46] Kevin Lynch argued that people who are unfamiliar with environments tend to orientate themselves by means of mental maps. People understand spaces through recognisable elements that provide legibility and emotional security of being in familiar territory. As a wayfinding designer, my aim is to provide users with that security. A good experience makes people feel supported and satisfied and engenders trust in that organisation. The result is a type of 'emotional wellness'. Conversely, a bad experience results in stress, discomfort and anxiety, resulting in frustration and erosion of trust in that institution. Establishing a clear mental map is a powerful aid in counteracting disorientation. Lynch proposed that these mental maps are formed by five key elements: paths, edges, districts, nodes and landmarks. So how does this apply to designing wayfinding systems?

When designing wayfinding systems, particularly for hospitals, we always ensure that paths you want people to travel along are clearly and easily understood. The analogy of a good butler with respect to corridors as described by Sonit Bafna and Julie Zook can be applied to a signage and wayfinding system that assists both visitors and staff in getting around a hospital. If the corridors are the butler, the signage is the butler's voice. The end goal of a wayfinding system is to get a person from location A to location B in the least disruptive and most stress-free method possible. In the context of a hospital, some visitors may be in a heightened state of stress, as such, the user-experience must be taken into consideration.

In the example below for the Northern Beaches Hospital in Sydney, we developed a wayfinding system that strongly signalled the key paths that people need to follow. We worked with photographer Tim Jones to create distinctly coloured wall graphics that functioned as intuitive wayfinding elements and that harmonised with the colours used in the interiors and furnishings.

It is also important to signal the edges of various zones as they play an organising role in defining the perimeter of an area. Creating distinct districts that have recognisable identifying characteristics is a powerful tool in orientation. It is also critical to develop the wayfinding system such that it reads as a uniform and hierarchical family of forms that are consistent in layout, typography, iconography and colour.

Nodal points in an environment are the best places to deliver information because these are where people pause to make decisions. The example in Figure 4.11 shows how we located both level and entire hospital directories at a key nodal point at the entry to a set of elevators. Access to various departments was accessible only through certain lift lobbies. Visitors therefore needed to be directed to the correct lobby.

The final key element touted by Lynch was creating landmark expressions in an environment to create points of reference that people can use to orientate themselves. On the Northern Beaches Hospital project, we collaborated with local artists and schools to develop the major graphic expression in the atrium space. It spans the balustrade of all seven floors in the atrium and is immediately visible when entering the

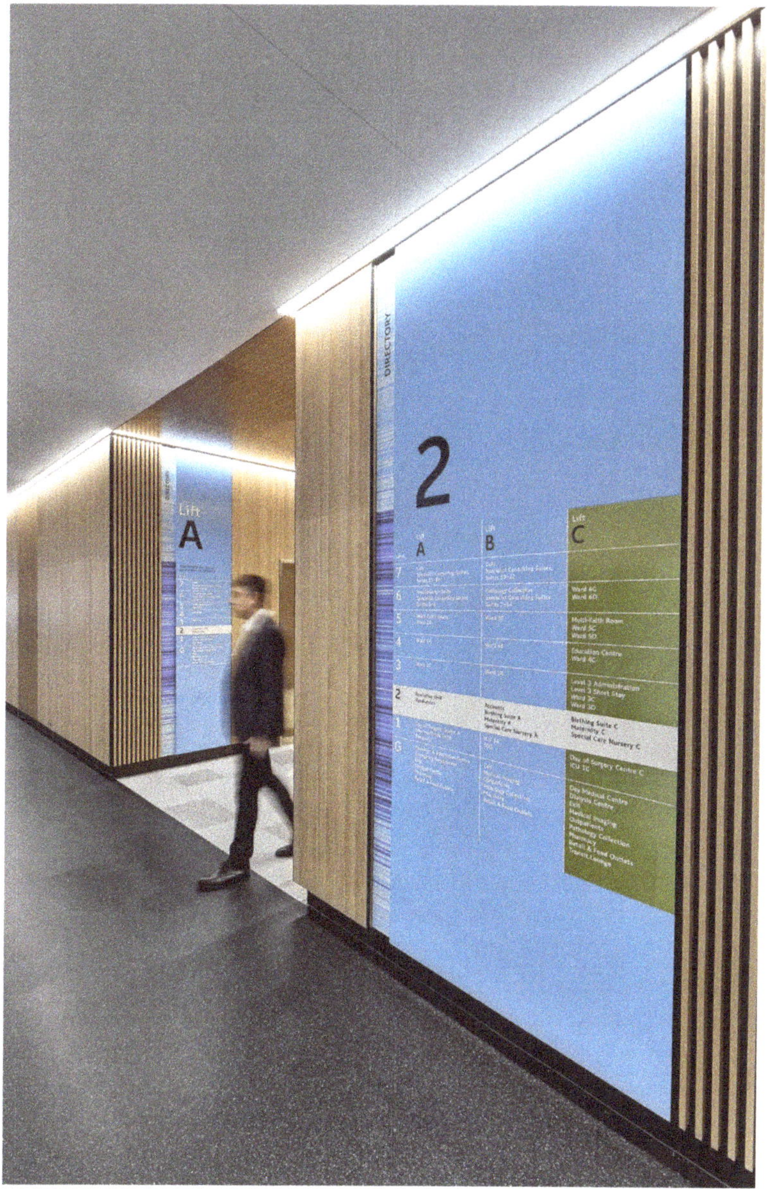

4.11 Northern Beaches Hospital level directories located at key nodal points. Copyright: Toby Peet.

front door of the hospital. This is shown below in Figure 4.12. We also employed environmental graphics at key destination points in the hospital to provide an intuitive layer to the wayfinding.

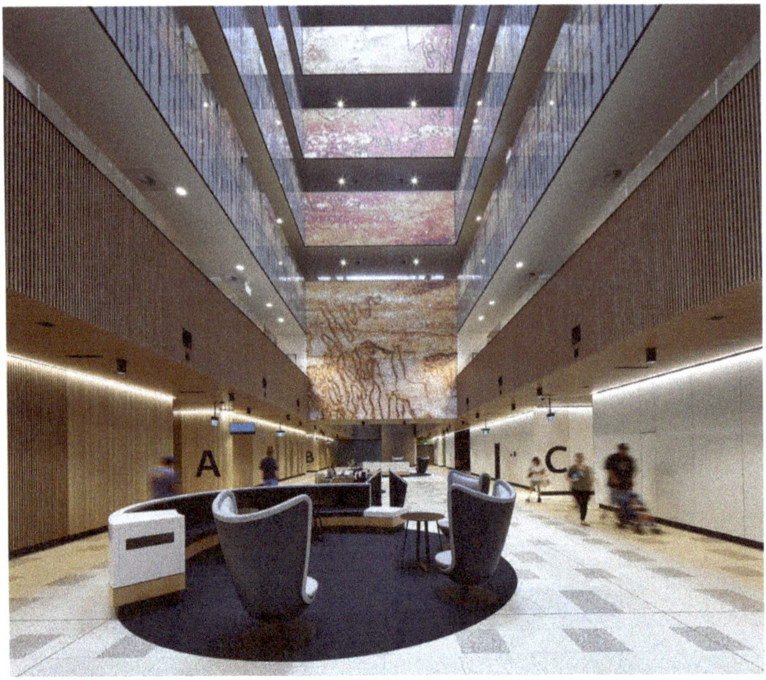

4.12 Northern Beaches Hospital atrium graphic. Copyright: Toby Peet.

When designing wayfinding systems, we need to understand how we can employ all these five key elements to develop more effective solutions. They all work together to create a more complete picture of the environment that visitors are navigating. In addition to Lynch's approach to developing wayfinding models, we often reference David Gibson's *The Wayfinding Handbook*.[47] In it, Gibson describes the four typical models that are seen in great cities around the world. These various models are employed to make the cities more comprehensible to users. The first is the 'connector model', exemplified by The Forbidden City in Beijing. This city is characterised by a strong central axis and a concentric system of gateways that clearly lead the way. The second is the 'districts model', after Cambridge. This is a city that has evolved organically over many centuries and has adopted individual precincts with distinct names, coats of arms and specific gateways. The third is the 'landmarks model', after Rome. This ancient city has axial roads and landmark focal points located at the centre point of each intersection and are major civic landmarks. Finally, the 'streets model', found in New York City, employs a simple wayfinding mechanism of a sequentially numbered grid of streets.

We often adopt one of these four models when planning signage and wayfinding systems for complex public buildings, depending on which is most relevant to the structure and layout of the architecture. Sometimes, we use a combination of models if we believe it will make the comprehension of the space more digestible.

In my view, one of the most important aspects of the creative process is to seek to uncover what is truly unique about a project. On the Northern Beaches Hospital, we developed a solution that was original and drew inspiration from the surrounding environment. The Hospital is located in Sydney's northern suburbs and is nestled between the beach and the bush. The surrounding natural environment provided rich sources of inspiration to the architects and interior designers.

We wanted to capture the essence of the place in our work as well, so we set off one weekend into the nearby national park in search of inspiration and returned with a few bags full of leaves, seed pods and various other items. Photographer Tim Jones captured them all in minute detail. The result of this is seen in the images in Figure 4.13.

We then coloured them to harmonise with the interior design scheme and applied them as environmental graphics throughout the building to assist with intuitive wayfinding. The graphics were intended

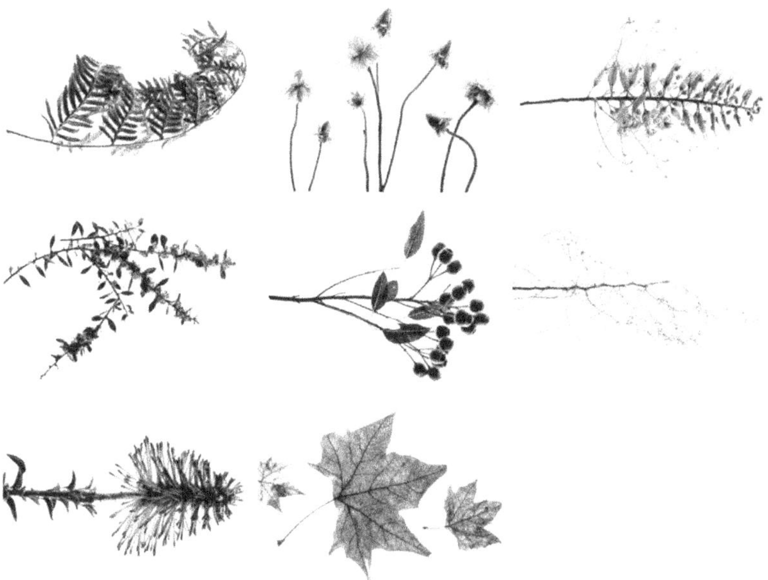

4.13 Original photography created for the environmental graphics. Copyright: Tim Jones.

to not only soothe the patients and visitors, but to activate the spaces, particularly long corridors and department check-ins.

The final two stages of the HCD process are prototyping our designs and then testing them to see whether they work. Prototyping can take many forms. We initially produce what we call 'lo-fi' prototypes and test them on-site to ensure that they work. This is a critical part of the HCD process, which enables us to iterate and improve the design where required. We also use 3D rendering software to prototype and test our designs. This allows us to produce very realistic renders of complex designs making it easy to see what the end-product will look like. It also makes it easy for the client to imagine what they are going to get, resulting in shorter approval times. The advent of 3D printing is making it easier to prototype scale models of our work. Complex designs can be created quickly and inexpensively. We also regularly produce 'hi-fi' prototypes. These are full size samples made of the actual materials that we have specified. We test these with users and modify the design if required.

Three takeaways

There are three key takeaways from adopting our creative design process to design wayfinding systems. First, seek to truly understand the audience that will engage with your work. Second, strive to uncover what is unique about your project and make that what drives the design outcome. And finally, prototype and test your work with your audience and learn from them. Following this prescribed approach maximises the opportunity to develop a solution that is more finely tuned to users' needs. I trust that this has given you some insight into our design methodology and how you can apply HCD to create more effective wayfinding systems.

Notes

1 Geoffrey M. Hodgson, 'What are institutions?', *Journal of Economic Issues*, 40, no. 1 (2006), 1–25.
2 Mary Douglas, *How Institutions Think* (New York: Syracuse University Press, 1986).
3 Thomas A. Markus, *Buildings and Power: Freedom and Control in the Origins of the Modern Building Type* (London: Routledge, 1993).
4 Clifford Whittingham Beers, *A Mind that Found Itself: An Autobiography* (Project Gutenberg Press, 1908/2004).
5 Erving Goffman, *The Presentation of Self in Everyday Life* (1st edition) (New York NY: Anchor, 1959).
6 Yelp: https://www.yelp.com/.
7 The history of European hospitals is full of examples of everyday life and medical care overlapping in intense ways, such as in Thompson and Goldin's account of the medieval hospital in Bruges. The sense of scandal about co-located activities, indicated by the Yelp

reviewers, can be traced back to Florence Nightingale. Not only did separation support the cleanliness that she aimed to embed architecturally, but she also sought to rescue nursing, as a profession, from association with prostitution. Eric M. 'never saw something like' flirtatious nurses or simultaneous suffering and partying in his life because hospital arrangements that allowed such things were largely phased out in the Victorian era. John D. Thompson and Grace Goldin, *The Hospital: A Social and Architectural History* (New Haven CT and London: Yale University Press, 1975).

Reconnecting the realms of normal social activity and healthcare is increasingly an overt goal of community-based clinics aimed at building population health in the United States. While Maggie's Centres aim to connect life and health through compelling architectural design, they generally house social spaces, not medical ones.

8 Edward C. Tolman, 'Cognitive maps in rats and men', *Psychological Review*, 55, no. 4 (1948), 189–208.

9 This distinction emerged quite early. An influential reference is R. A. Hart and G. T. Moore, 'The development of spatial cognition: a review', in Roger M. Downs and David Stea (eds), *Image and Environment: Cognitive Mapping and Spatial Behavior* (Chicago IL: Aldine Pub Co, 1973), 246–88.

10 We say 'type of geometrical knowledge', to acknowledge that the geometrical relationships need not be entirely Euclidean, but could be just topological, such as knowing that some landmark is *within* a district, or that a room is *to the right* of a corridor.

11 Reginald G. Golledge, Valerie Dougherty and Scott Bell, 'Acquiring spatial knowledge: survey versus route-based knowledge in unfamiliar environments', *Annals of the Association of American Geographers*, 85, no. 1 (1995), 136. Note, Golledge and his colleagues speak of an *ability* of treating survey knowledge as *if* it is a map, and do not claim the existence of an actual map being represented in our head. But the description is still suggestive enough to wash out any subtle distinction that may be maintained between the two positions. The warning against taking cognitive map as a literal mental map is made quite explicitly in Alexander W. Siegel and Sheldon H. White, 'The development of spatial representations of large-scale environments', in Hayne W. Reese (ed.), *Advances in Child Development and Behavior*, vol. 10 (JAI, 1975), 9–55, a paper that is cited in Golledge *et al.*

12 Hart and Moore, 'Development of spatial cognition', and Siegel and White, 'Development of spatial representations' (both cited above) are both influential accounts of this view. The point-line-plane order that informs this view was widespread at the time; it also guided Kevin Lynch's framework for the mental organisation of the city's image: *The Image of the City* (Cambridge MA: MIT Press, 1960). Montello, in 'A new framework' (cited below) provides a useful contextualisation of the emergence of this idea.

13 For instance, Christoph Hölscher *et al.* ('Up the down staircase: wayfinding strategies in multi-level buildings', *Journal of Environmental Psychology*, 26, no. 4 (1 December 2006), 284–99), saw fit to cast their study as a comparison between their subjects' survey and route knowledge and judged the quality of survey knowledge through a pointing test, treating this kind of knowledge, in effect, as an act of visualising a mental map.

14 Paul Arthur and Romedi Passini, *Wayfinding: People, Signs, and Architecture* (Ontario, Canada: Focus Strategic Communications, 2002), 108–10. Originally published in 1992 by McGraw Hill, the book introduced the term 'wayfinding' as an integrated design problem.

15 Arthur and Passini, *Wayfinding*, 109–10.

16 Shannon Dawn Moeser, 'Cognitive mapping in a complex building', *Environment and Behavior*, 20, no. 1 (1 January 1988), 21–49.

17 Unless they have been trained to work with maps. Golledge *et al.*, 'Acquiring spatial knowledge'.

18 Hölscher *et al.*, 'Up the down staircase'.

19 The core site of this mapping is the hippocampus – a distinctively shaped sub-cortical formation of neural tissue that sits just under the temporal cortex of the brain. The hippocampus receives connections from various cortical regions and has neural projections to a few specific areas of the temporal cortex. This work has been reported by a large number of papers, but the following two publications provide a nicely contextualised and comprehensive description of the research work and its findings: John O'Keefe and Lynn Nadel, *The Hippocampus as a Cognitive Map* (Oxford and New York: Oxford University Press, 1978); and, John O'Keefe, 'Kant and the Sea-Horse: an essay in the neurophilosophy of space', in Naomi Eilan, Rosaleen McCarthy and Bill Brewer (eds), *Spatial Representation* (Cambridge: Blackwell, 1993).

20 The work of O'Keefe and his colleagues is concerned with the vertebrate brain in general; much of the basic research has been done on mice, but it has also been extended to humans.

21 Coding information in this way is not sufficient for the animal to develop a completely allocentric knowledge of the environment. O'Keefe ('Kant and the Sea Horse', 58–9) discusses a set of criteria that would need to be satisfied by a spatial navigational system before an entirely allocentric knowledge of the environment could be said to have been achieved, but the mechanism by which these criteria could be met remain to be explicated.

22 O'Keefe and his colleagues have conducted a few studies to understand the role of the hippocampus in the learned knowledge of building layouts among human subjects: see, for example, Eleanor A. Maguire *et al.*, 'Knowing where and getting there: a human navigation network', *Science*, 280, no. 5365 (1998), 921–4. But, while these studies have confirmed the role of the hippocampus in the creation and maintenance of spatial memory, they have not added further to our understanding of the way knowledge of entire layouts is stored in the mind.

23 This point explains the finding (discussed above) of people being able to navigate successfully within an environment, but not being able to draw a map of it or to locate various places of interest on a given map. Also, because the use of the map-as-sensor depends on the mostly visual recognition of cues from within a setting, a person may learn an environment through cues encountered in one orientation (as visitors moving through a new building often do) but may fail to recognise the same set of cues when viewing them from a different direction (as in a return trip) and so may become lost. This point also explains how long-time residents of a city, who can navigate it successfully as they go about their day-to-day lives, may nevertheless fail to recognise settings when shown photographs of them – a point that Kevin Lynch reports in his study of what makes cities memorable (*cf. Image of the City*, cited above).

24 The work of Barbara Tversky is particularly cogent on this point. Useful summaries can be found in Barbara Tversky, 'Cognitive maps, cognitive collages, and spatial mental models', in Andrew U. Frank and Irene Campari (eds), *Spatial Information Theory: A Theoretical Basis for GIS: Lecture Notes in Computer Science* (Berlin, Heidelberg: Springer, 1993), 14–24; and in, Barbara Tversky, 'Structures of mental spaces: how people think about space', *Environment and Behavior*, 35, no. 1 (1 January 2003), 66–80.

25 We use the term 'mental model' circumspectly in the narrow sense advocated by Lance Rips (in 'Mental muddles', in Myles Brand and Robert M. Harnish (eds), *The Representation of Knowledge and Belief*, Arizona Colloquium in Cognition (Tucson AZ: University of Arizona Press, 1986), 258–86), that is, without committing to the larger idea that mental models provide the framework for our cognitive ability as a whole. This latter idea has been advocated classically by P. N. Johnson-Laird, *Mental Models: Towards a Cognitive Science of Language, Inference and Consciousness* (Cambridge and New York: Cambridge University Press, 1983). We should also acknowledge that the conception of cognitive maps as mental models is not a new one (see our citations of Tversky's work above).

26 It is a feature of this system that it allows us to navigate autonomously without being aware of what we are doing, as when we sometimes find that we have arrived at a place with almost no memory of journey.

27 We use the term 'system' somewhat loosely to speak about the range of spatial problem-solving abilities that support navigation as a collective, but without meaning to suggest that a dedicated single system exists for this purpose.

28 Steffen Werner, Bernd Krieg-Brückner and Theo Herrmann, 'Modelling navigational knowledge by route graphs', *Lecture Notes in Computer Science: Spatial Cognition II – Integrating Abstract Theories, Empirical Studies, Formal Methods, and Practical Applications* (2000), 295.

29 Edward K. Sadalla and Daniel R. Montello, 'Remembering changes in direction', *Environment and Behavior*, 21, no. 3 (1989), 346–63.

30 Daniel R. Montello, 'Spatial orientation and the angularity of urban routes: a field-study', *Environment and Behavior*, 23, no. 1 (1991), 47–69.

31 Sadalla and Montello, 'Remembering changes in direction'.

32 Integration can be roughly indexed by the average turns that separate any given corridor from all other corridors.

33 John Peponis, Craig Zimring and Yoon Kyung Choi, 'Finding the building in wayfinding', *Environment and Behavior*, 22, no. 5 (1 September 1990), 555–90. The drawings show the plan of the building studied and a diagram that represents the network of corridors as a set of straight-line segments. The study found that the degree of integration of the corridors was

highly correlated (r=0.757, p<0.1). The researchers also found that corridor crossings on higher integrated corridors were visited far more than those on less integrated corridors by subjects during the directed search (r=0.778, p<0.1).

34 Saif Haq, 'Investigating the syntax line: configurational properties and cognitive correlates', *Environment and Planning B: Planning and Design*, 30, no. 6 (1 December 2003): 841–63; also reported in Saif Haq and Craig Zimring, 'Just down the road a piece: the development of topological knowledge of building layouts', *Environment and Behavior*, 35 (1 January 2003), 132–60.

35 We use the term 'institution' broadly to refer to settled and relatively permanent forms of collective behaviour that have been established through social norms. For the classical definition, see Everett C. Hughes, 'The ecological aspect of institutions', *American Sociological Review*, 1, no. 2 (1936), 180–9. Building types are institutions because they are shaped around established patterns of behaviour governed by social norms; in hospitals such behavioural norms are quite strong and even coercive, at least in their core programmatic areas.

36 For a focused description of institutional types in architecture, see Julia Robinson, *Institution and Home: Architecture as Cultural Medium* (Delft: Techne Press, 2006), 204.

37 An institutional form that is best described in Mary Douglas's useful formulation as high grid, given that hospital settings are by definition also a strong group type. The original account of the ideas is in Mary Douglas, *Natural Symbols: Explorations in Cosmology* (London: Random House, 1970).

38 Roger G. Barker and Phil Schoggen, *Qualities of Community Life: Methods of Measuring Environment and Behavior Applied to an American and an English Town* (San Francisco CA: Jossey-Bass, 1973).

39 See Mary Douglas, *How Institutions Think: The Frank W. Abrams Lectures* (Syracuse NY: Syracuse University Press, 1986). Douglas makes a forceful case for the necessity of collective thought to maintain institutions, arguing that such thought creates classificatory schemes on which institutional practice is based, and that classificatory schemes are based on naturalised analogies understood by all participants of the institutions.

40 David Cohn, 'Maternity and pediatric hospital, *Architectural Record* (1 October 2004), 156–61. The short description can be found on the journal website at https://www.architecturalrecord.com/articles/12143-maternity-and-pediatric-hospital.

41 And this is by deliberate design, as we learn from the architect's own text: 'This project is another good example of the role the floor plan has played in architectural practice, for it is the layout of this floor plan that influences the complex program of a hospital in which each ward is a building block. The concatenation of wards gives way to courtyards that can and must be considered characteristic elements of this project, as providing the patients with a comfortable environment was one of the architect's goals. Such comfort is also achieved through the choice of materials both inside and out, which seek to be perceived as indicative of a technological culture to which a hospital is no stranger. Clarity, cleanliness, and brightness are attributes of hygiene and also of this architecture, which we would like to describe as rational and optimistic.' Rafael Moneo, 'Hospital Materno-Infantil Gregorio Marañón. En Colaboración Con José María de La Mata Madrid, España', Rafael Moneo Arquitecto, n.d., https://rafaelmoneo.com/en/projects/maternity-and-pediatrics-hospital-of-gregorio-maranon-hospital (accessed 13 August 2021).

42 A well-known argument in favour of this point is in Nelson Goodman, 'When is art?', in David Perkins and Barbara Leondar (eds), *The Arts and Cognition* (Baltimore MD: Johns Hopkins University Press, 1977). However, the most sustained defence of the idea that an interaction with a clear contextual history is all that is needed to separate a work of art from its physically indistinguishable counterpart is found in the work of Arthur Danto. The standard reference for this idea is Arthur C. Danto, *The Transfiguration of the Commonplace: A Philosophy of Art* (reprint edition) (Cambridge MA: Harvard University Press, 1983).

43 This perspective on museums draws on Eilean Hooper-Greenhill, *Museums and the Shaping of Knowledge* (London: Routledge, 1992).

44 This study has a very small sample size but is a good example of an early video-based intervention aimed at pain reduction: A. C. Miller, L. C. Hickman and G. K. Lemasters, 'A distraction technique for control of burn pain', *The Journal of Burn Care and Rehabilitation*, 13 (1992), 576–80. The most influential study of the role of aesthetics of views on health outcomes remains Roger Ulrich, 'View through a window may influence recovery from surgery', *Science*, 224 (1984), 420–1. A summary on evidence-based design research on hospital art appears in

Kathy Hathorn and Upali Nanda, 'A guide to evidence-based art' (Center for Health Design, 2008). More recent studies have larger sample sizes, and some have replaced pain-related outcome variables with measurements of satisfaction.

45 Ben Lerner's nameless protagonist describes just this situation in the short story 'The Golden Vanity'. Ben Lerner, 'The Golden Vanity', *New Yorker* (18 July 2012), https://www.newyorker.com/magazine/2012/06/18/the-golden-vanity.

46 Kevin Lynch, *The Image of the City* (Boston MA: The MIT Press, 1960).

47 David Gibson, *The Wayfinding Handbook* (Princeton NJ: Princeton Architectural Press, 2009).

References

Arthur, Paul, and Romedi Passini, *Wayfinding: People, Signs, and Architecture* (Ontario, Canada: Focus Strategic Communications, 2002).

Barker, Roger G., and Phil Schoggen, *Qualities of Community Life: Methods of Measuring Environment and Behavior Applied to an American and an English Town* (San Francisco CA: Jossey-Bass, 1973).

Cohn, David, 'Maternity and pediatric hospital', *Architectural Record*, 10 (1 October 2004), 156–61, https://www.architecturalrecord.com/articles/12143-maternity-and-pediatric-hospital.

Danto, Arthur C., *The Transfiguration of the Commonplace: A Philosophy of Art* (reprint edition) (Cambridge MA: Harvard University Press, 1983).

Douglas, Mary, *Natural Symbols: Explorations in Cosmology* (London: Random House, 1970).

Douglas, Mary, *How Institutions Think* (New York: Syracuse University Press, 1986).

Gibson, David. *The Wayfinding Handbook* (Princeton NJ: Princeton Architectural Press, 2009).

Goffman, Erving, *The Presentation of Self in Everyday Life* (Harmondsworth: Penguin Books, 1959).

Goffman, Erving, *Interaction Ritual: Essays on Face-to-Face Behavior* (Garden City NY: Doubleday, 1967).

Golledge, Reginald G., Valerie Dougherty and Scott Bell, 'Acquiring spatial knowledge: survey versus route-based knowledge in unfamiliar environments', *Annals of the Association of American Geographers*, 85, no. 1 (1995), 134–58.

Goodman, Nelson, 'When is art?', in David Perkins and Barbara Leondar (eds), *The Arts and Cognition* (Baltimore MD: Johns Hopkins University Press, 1977).

Haq, Saif, 'Investigating the syntax line: configurational properties and cognitive correlates', *Environment and Planning B: Planning and Design*, 30, no. 6 (2003), 841–63.

Haq, Saif, and Craig Zimring, 'Just down the road a piece: the development of topological knowledge of building layouts', *Environment and Behavior*, 35, no. 1 (2003), 132–60.

Hart, R. A., and G. T. Moore, 'The development of spatial cognition: a review', in Roger M. Downs and David Stea (eds), *Image and Environment: Cognitive Mapping and Spatial Behavior* (Chicago IL: Aldine Pub Co, 1973), 246–88.

Hathorn, Kathy, and Upali Nanda, 'A guide to evidence-based art' (Center for Health Design, 2008).

Hodgson, Geoffrey M., 'What are institutions?', *Journal of Economic Issues*, 40, no. 1 (2006), 1–25.

Hölscher, Christoph, *et al.*, 'Up the down staircase: wayfinding strategies in multi-level buildings', *Journal of Environmental Psychology*, 26, no. 4 (1 December 2006), 284–99.

Hooper-Greenhill, Eilean, *Museums and the Shaping of Knowledge* (London: Routledge, 1992).

Hughes, Everett C., 'The ecological aspect of institutions', *American Sociological Review*, 1, no. 2 (1936), 180–9.

Johnson-Laird, P. N., *Mental Models: Towards a Cognitive Science of Language, Inference and Consciousness* (Cambridge and New York: Cambridge University Press, 1983).

Lerner, Ben, 'The Golden Vanity', *New Yorker* (18 July 2012), https://www.newyorker.com/magazine/2012/06/18/the-golden-vanity.

Lynch, Kevin, *The Image of the City* (Boston MA: The MIT Press, 1960).

Maguire, Eleanor A., *et al.*, 'Knowing where and getting there: a human navigation network', *Science*, 280, no. 5365 (1998), 921–4.

Markus, Thomas A., *Buildings and Power: Freedom and Control in the Origin of Modern Building Types* (London: Routledge, 1993).

Miller, A. C., L. C. Hickman and G. K. Lemasters, 'A distraction technique for control of burn pain', *The Journal of Burn Care and Rehabilitation*, 13 (1992), 576–80.

Moeser, Shannon Dawn, 'Cognitive mapping in a complex building', *Environment and Behavior*, 20, no. 1 (1988), 21–49.

Moneo, Rafael, 'Hospital Materno-Infantil Gregorio Marañón. En Colaboración Con José María de La Mata Madrid, España', Rafael Moneo Arquitecto, n.d., https://rafaelmoneo.com/en/projects/maternity-and-pediatrics-hospital-of-gregorio-maranon-hospital (accessed 13 August 2021).

Montello, Daniel R., 'Spatial orientation and the angularity of urban routes: a field-study', *Environment and Behavior*, 23, no. 1 (1991), 47–69.

O'Keefe, John, 'Kant and the Sea-Horse: an essay in the neurophilosophy of space', in Naomi Eilan, Rosaleen McCarthy and Bill Brewer (eds), *Spatial Representation: Problems in Philosophy and Psychology* (Cambridge: Blackwell, 1993), 43–64.

O'Keefe, John, and Lynn Nadel, *The Hippocampus as a Cognitive Map* (Oxford and New York: Oxford University Press, 1978).

Peponis, John, Craig Zimring and Yoon Kyung Choi, 'Finding the building in wayfinding', *Environment and Behavior*, 22, no. 5 (1990), 555–90. https://doi.org/10.1177/0013916590225001.

Rips, Lance, 'Mental muddles', in Myles Brand and Robert M. Harnish (eds), *The Representation of Knowledge and Belief* (Arizona Colloquium in Cognition) (Tucson AZ: University of Arizona Press, 1986), 258–86.

Robinson, Julia, *Institution and Home: Architecture as Cultural Medium* (Delft: Techne Press, 2006).

Sadalla, Edward K., and Daniel R. Montello, 'Remembering changes in direction', *Environment and Behavior*, 21, no. 3 (1989), 346–63.

Siegel, Alexander W., and Sheldon H. White, 'The development of spatial representations of large-scale environments', in Hayne W. Reese (ed.), *Advances in Child Development and Behavior*, vol. 10 (New York: Academic, JAI, 1975), 9–55.

Thompson, John D., and Grace Goldin, *The Hospital: A Social and Architectural History* (New Haven CT and London: Yale University Press, 1975).

Tolman, Edward C., 'Cognitive maps in rats and men', *Psychological Review*, 55, no. 4 (1948), 189–208.

Tversky, Barbara, 'Cognitive maps, cognitive collages, and spatial mental models', in Andrew U. Frank and Irene Campari (eds), *Spatial Information: Theory A Theoretical Basis for GIS: Lecture Notes in Computer Science* (Berlin, Heidelberg: Springer, 1993), 14–24.

Tversky, Barbara, 'Structures of mental spaces: how people think about space', *Environment and Behavior*, 35, no. 1 (2003), 66–80.

Ulrich, Roger, 'View through a window may influence recovery from surgery', *Science*, 224 (1984), 420–1.

Werner, Steffen, Bernd Krieg-Brückner and Theo Herrmann, 'Modelling navigational knowledge by route graphs', in C. Freska, C. Habel, W. Brauer and K. F. Wender (eds), *Spatial Cognition II: Lecture Notes in Computer Science* (Berlin, Heidelberg: Springer, 2000), 295–316.

Whittingham Beers, Clifford, *A Mind that Found Itself: An Autobiography* (Project Gutenberg Press, 1908/2004).

Chapter 5: Outlook
The social logic of spaces for health: The relational hospital as a response to COVID-19

Kerstin Sailer

As I am writing this in spring 2021, more than a year after the new Coronavirus SARS-CoV-2 (COVID) was detected and looking back to the different healthcare design responses to COVID with the advantages of today's knowledge and insight,[1] a story of variability and opportunity structures emerges. In this chapter I will argue that pandemic architecture can be read as a reflection of resources and possibilities available to different healthcare systems and governance structures around the world and highlight how that interpretation underlines the relevance of considering hospitals in their social logic and thus as relational structures.

Adapting spaces to emerging needs is of course a normal process, yet the urgency, immediacy and scale of what COVID required hospitals to do, was aptly described as a 'reinvention' by UK medical doctor Rachel Clarke during the first wave in spring 2020:

> The pandemic is the first nationwide major incident in NHS history … with no end in sight. Local teams across the country are working with urgency and passion to do whatever is needed to save as many lives as they can. Hospitals are reinventing themselves with astonishing alacrity. All non-urgent surgery is suspended, just as it would be in a local major incident. Operating theatres, recovery areas, normal wards and even conference rooms are transformed into ersatz ICUs.[2]

Normal protocols developed for major incidents seemed insufficient according to Clarke. Those usually include alerting staff, preparing emergency and intensive care departments, shifting mobile patients to other hospitals further afield and cancelling all elective operations for a few days in order to create surge capacity. Yet what turns out to be an efficient machinery for an isolated incident (such as a terrorist attack) does not necessarily cope in the same way with the challenges of a highly infectious new disease, spreading rapidly and continuously for many months.

The way in which buildings and their usage changed during the pandemic can be described as a continuation and acceleration of existing trends.[3] For example, the importance of infection control and the problem of hospital-acquired (nosocomial) infections was already on the agenda due to – among other factors – an increasing concern regarding antimicrobial resistance. COVID accelerated this issue, rendering the close monitoring of pathogen spread as highest priority.

In the following I will discuss the change in perspectives that the pandemic has enforced on us as a continuation and acceleration of previous trends and developments, as well as an opportunity to reflect on hospital design and what we can learn for the future. This means taking up Clarke's theme of reinvention, asking how we might want to reinvent hospital spaces for a post-pandemic era. In doing so, I aim to look forward by looking back, weaving in aspects discussed in the earlier chapters of this book, ranging from the way in which specialised building types emerge (Zook in Chapter 1), to concurrent aspects of patient oversight (Ossmann in Chapter 2), care team communication (Pachilova and Sailer in Chapter 3) and cognition and visitor wayfinding (Bafna and Zook in Chapter 4). I will also refer explicitly to the contributions made by the practitioner essays of this book.

Essentially, I want to argue that design is always a response to priorities, and as priorities shift and change – from an individual to a collective view of health, from local expertise to shared knowledge, from a technological approach to a primacy of social exchange and human touch – design must follow suit. But before we reflect on emerging priorities, let us delve more deeply into the pandemic and what we can learn from how we have coped with COVID.

Healthcare spaces in times of COVID

It might seem glaringly obvious to argue that health has become crucially important in times of a global pandemic; yet a very particular shift in perception and lived reality has occurred around the globe and that is the newly found focus on the importance of public health for economic, social and individual prosperity and wellbeing. Public health in this sense does not only include the idea of the healthiness of the overall population; for instance, in pre-pandemic times public health concerns focused, among other things, on sugar intake, access to nutritious food and levels of obesity across a nation or levels of exercise and fitness. What the pandemic has added is the idea of mutual influence. My health is also your health, if we share a common space, and, likewise, my precautionary behaviour during a pandemic (distancing, contact reduction, wearing a mask) not only protects me from harm, but also others around me. This understanding of the interdependence of public health moves the focus of attention away from the individual or certain groups of individuals (e.g., by demographics) onto relationships and connections.[4]

Alongside the renaissance of public health, interior healthcare spaces also received more attention than usual from architects and planners. Hospitals around the world underwent a whole range of extensions, transformations and spatial as well as organisational reinventions. Researchers have identified four different strategies for how the physical fabric of hospitals was altered or extended due to COVID:

1. transforming non-healthcare spaces (e.g., sports facilities, exhibition centres and car parks);
2. transforming hospital spaces, including benign changes such as coloured markings on floors to demarcate areas, using new signage, installing Plexiglas walls or using multiple entrances to hospitals where possible, as well as all the way to larger interventions, such as installing triage spaces at the entrance, sealing off doors to change navigation and movement flow patterns, repurposing operating theatres and turning them into ICU wards;
3. creating plug-in spaces to existing hospitals; and
4. implementing insights into ongoing architectural design projects.[5]

It cannot be denied how starkly responses differed across countries, also depending on how hard and how early they were hit by COVID. A more detailed and contextualised account of two countries reacting to the pandemic challenges in very different ways can shine a spotlight on further architectural or spatial strategies and, as such, will be presented in the next two sections, focusing on China and the United Kingdom.

Chinese hospital spaces in context

By the end of December 2019,[6] doctors in China had become alarmed by a cluster of atypical pneumonia cases in the Wuhan region. It was reported to the World Health Organization, identified as a novel coronavirus on 9 January 2020 and in the following weeks human-to-human transmission was confirmed. On 23 January 2020, during the Chinese Spring Festival celebrations, travel and movement restrictions were issued in several Chinese cities – at that time, China had reported 571 cases and 17 deaths.

As of late March 2021, more than 15 months after its discovery, fewer than 5,000 total deaths[7] have been associated with COVID in China, a remarkably low figure given what we know today of the viral spread of the disease.

Experts argued that China's rapid response, its rigorous testing regime, surveillance mechanisms (e.g., temperature checks), a hard and swift lockdown, as well as high compliance in the population (e.g., wearing masks or staying at home) allowed segregating COVID cases from the healthy population, thus keeping the overall case count and mortality figures relatively low.[8]

In addition, the way in which hospital spaces were configured, built and used in China also contributed to this success story. Three architectural strategies are worth pointing out.

First, hospitals in a city or a region worked together, allowing some hospitals to quickly specialise in the care for COVID patients, while transferring non-respiratory medical cases to other hospitals in the same municipality. With this simple move, nosocomial infections were kept to a minimum.

Second, in the epicentre of the outbreak – the region of Wuhan, but also in other provinces with an early clustering of cases – additional standalone makeshift hospitals were purpose-built. Most prominently, the Huoshenshan (Fire God Mountain) hospital (1,000 beds) and the Leishenshan (Thunder God Mountain) hospital (1,500 beds) were constructed in Wuhan in the very short period of just 10 days. Planners were able to draw on insights derived from the construction of the Xiaotangshan hospital in Beijing, erected during the SARS outbreak in 2003, where none of its 1,383 medical workers became infected.[9] The hospitals consisted of a series of prefabricated containers installed on site. Their spatial logic (see Figure 5.1) is intrinsically characterised by strict infection control, separation of flows and modularity: patients are accommodated in double-bed rooms with en-suite bathrooms, enclosed on all sides. Fifty beds form one medical unit (in a wing, see Figures 5.2

and 5.3) and four medical units work together as a medical zone. Nursing staff enter the unit through a central double-loaded corridor and can enter patient rooms from there via an anteroom, servicing two rooms to either side. A separate and unconnected corridor loops around the outside of a wing, available to patients. This is also accessible from the outside to bring patients in or out. Nurses leave the unit through a series of separate rooms, where they can peel out of their layers of protective personal equipment (PPE). Therefore, the configuration strictly separates areas considered clean in the central spine; areas considered semi-contaminated (i.e., the double-loaded corridors in each unit available to nursing staff); and contaminated areas (i.e., the patient rooms and U-shaped corridor looping around the unit).

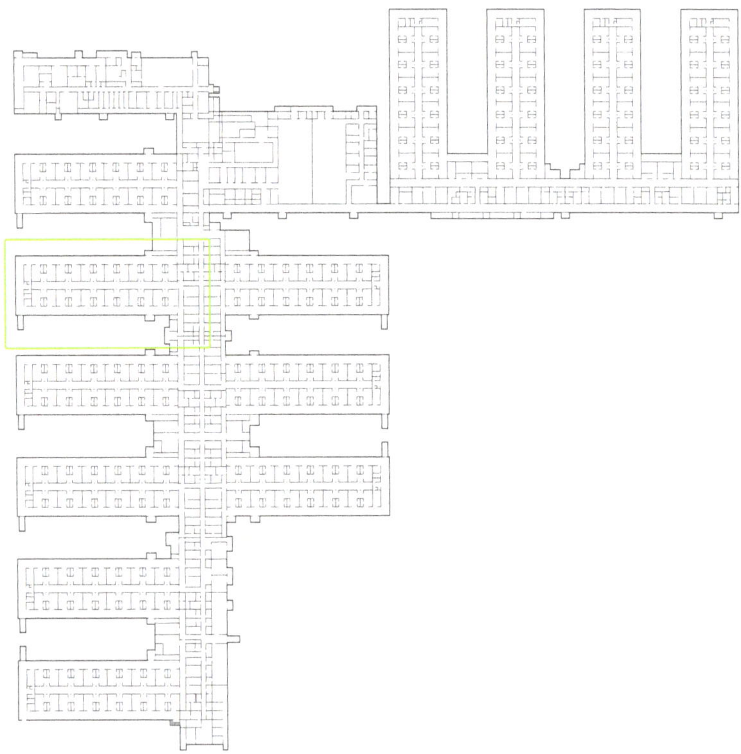

5.1 Floorplan of the Huoshenshan mobile hospital in Wuhan, erected in 2020. Plan redrawn by Victor Carrillo and Daniel Rios, 2021.

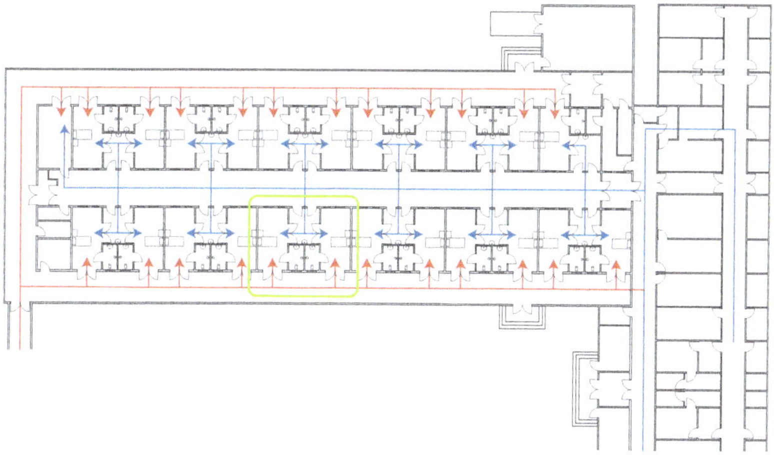

5.2 The ward with separate circulation loops for nurses and patients at the Huoshenshan hospital. Plan redrawn by Victor Carrillo and Daniel Rios, 2021.

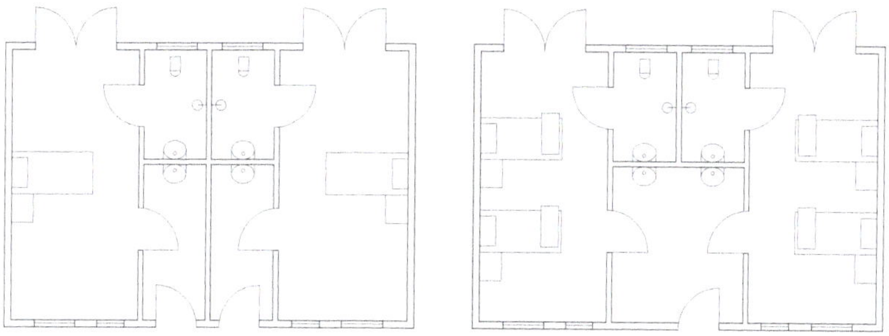

5.3 Suspected cases are isolated, while confirmed cases are cohorted. Plan redrawn by Victor Carrillo and Daniel Rios, 2021.

Third, a different type of hospital was provided, repurposing existing infrastructures such as large sports halls or conference centres to accommodate patients who tested positive for COVID, yet only displayed mild symptoms – the so-called 'Fangcang shelter hospitals' (see Figure 5.4). These hospitals provided a network of 16 buildings in the Wuhan region offering 13,000 beds[10] and allowing a temporary separation of infected people from their families, friends and neighbours to limit cross-infections and the psychological stress involved for all. In addition to enabling strategic isolation and triaging of patients according to the severity of symptoms, the Fangcang shelters also provided basic medical care,

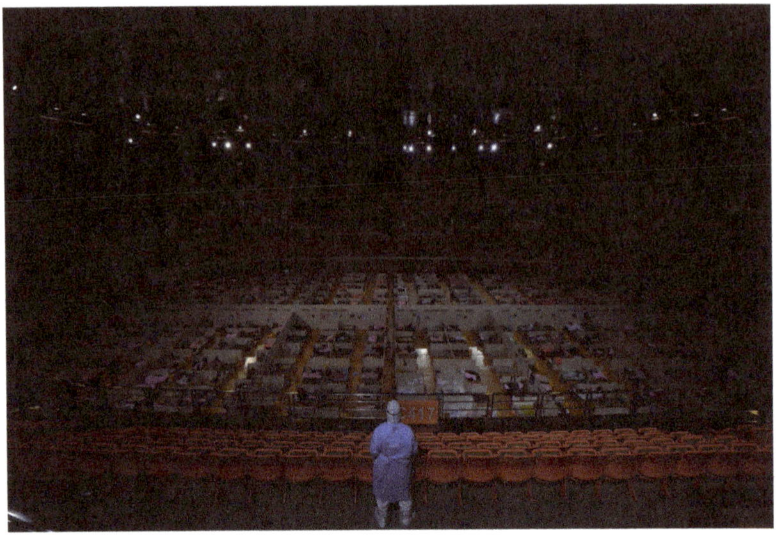

5.4 A Fangcang shelter hospital erected in the Wuhan Sports Centre. Copyright: Wang Jing.

mental-health counselling and a quick referral system for patients with worsening conditions.[11] Accommodating mostly fit and mobile adults, the spatial structure was designed with a focus on community, socialisation and recuperation. Beds were tightly packed in the large open halls of the shelters, allowing 1.5 metres between beds and curtains on two sides, which were drawn back most of the time (Figure 5.4). Female and male wards were separated, and activity spaces were provided either side for eating, exercise, group reading, dancing, etc. While patients perceived some deprivation of their privacy, they also felt solidarity, equality and a sense of camaraderie, according to interviews undertaken alongside a detailed space syntax analysis of the spatial structure, provided by Li *et al.*[12]

In summary, a sophisticated and nuanced architectural and spatial strategy based on high-level triaging and tailored makeshift designs contributed to China's effective management of COVID.

UK hospital spaces in context

The first confirmed case of a COVID-19 infection was reported in the United Kingdom on 1 February 2020.[13] As of late March 2021, a bit more than a year later, an excess of 125,000 people have died from COVID in the United Kingdom, constituting one of the highest death rates per inhabitant in the world.[14]

Despite having witnessed the strict and early lockdown in China, as well as overwhelmed healthcare systems in Northern Italy where COVID first took hold in Europe, the UK government initially reacted reservedly, not recognising the dangers fully and communicating mixed messages,[15] while also allowing large-scale events such as the horse racing at the Cheltenham Festival to go ahead in early March 2020.

This led to a quick rise in cases (although the majority in the first wave of March and April 2020 remained untested), followed by increasing hospitalisations and deaths and, in turn, an enormous pressure on the National Health Service (NHS), as well as individual hospitals faced with making decisions locally at speed and scale. The degree to which hospitals adapted to the surge of patients remains undocumented, but it can be safely assumed that every single hospital underwent at least benign changes and adaptations, such as shifting functionalities and creating extra capacity, as outlined by Rachel Clarke in her book *Breath Taking* and highlighted at the beginning of the chapter.

An audio diary from one NHS hospital, the Bradford Royal Infirmary, provides another first-hand account of how the situation evolved in the early days of the pandemic:

> Since my visit four days ago, the ward has moved quickly from having a few cases isolated in side-rooms to the whole ward being full of COVID-positive cases.
>
> (Bradford Royal Infirmary, 8 April 2020)[16]

> The hospital has metamorphosed from a complex galaxy of specialities to a single planet of COVID-19. We are coping well with the surge, but there is so much we still don't know about this new and deadly virus.
>
> (Bradford Royal Infirmary, 22 April 2020)[17]

> [It's the] 5th of May. The Head of the NHS has written to all hospitals in the UK setting out his ambition to return to normal by six weeks' time. It's a goal we all support, but it feels a little disconnected from what is happening at the COVID coal face. Patients continue to knock at our hospital door in steady and relentless numbers.
>
> (Bradford Royal Infirmary, 13 May 2020)[18]

The three quotes by medical doctor and professor John Wright paint a similar picture to the one described by Rachel Clarke of increasing numbers of COVID patients coming in and first taking over side rooms, then whole wards, before engulfing the majority of the hospital. Contrary to the examples presented from China, a strict separation of regular patients and confirmed COVID cases did not succeed, also due to the unavailability of tests. Instead, attempts to triage were made inside hospitals as best as possible, for instance by floor markings, visually separating respiratory (COVID) and non-respiratory emergency department spaces. Turning whole hospitals into dedicated places for COVID care as seen in China was only taken up in the second UK wave of COVID in December 2020.[19] In addition, there was no place for patients with a mild course of disease, or in fact COVID positive patients well enough to leave hospital, which meant they were sent back home including to care homes, therefore seeding COVID among the most vulnerable populations.[20] A lack of resources, including PPE, led to a high rate of nosocomial infections among healthcare workers.[21]

Similar to responses in other countries, the spatial strategy of refurbishing existing infrastructure was also employed in the United Kingdom, creating spare capacity by erecting standalone new hospital structures (i.e., the NHS Nightingale hospitals, named after nursing pioneer Florence Nightingale). Large conference or exhibition centres such as the London ExCel or the Glasgow SEC were transformed into open-plan wards in the Nightingale tradition, designed by architecture practice BDP (see Figure 5.5).[22]

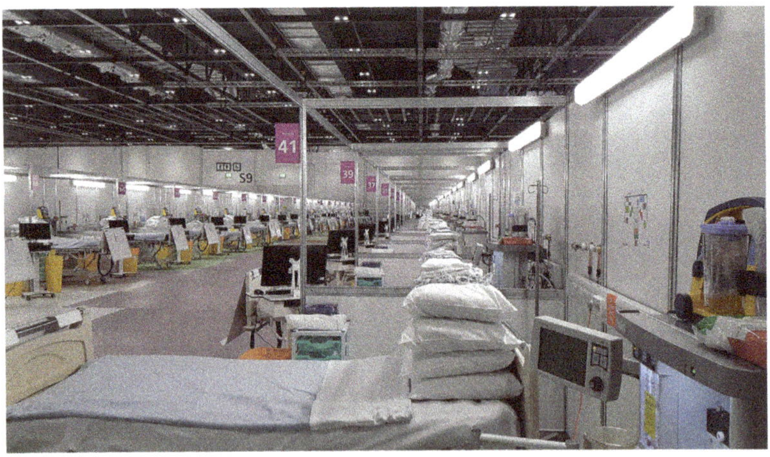

5.5 NHS Nightingale hospital designed by BDP. Image courtesy of BDP.

Within a short time, thousands of extra beds, mostly in intensive care were created across the country, marking an unprecedented effort of the UK construction industry, supported by the military. The design principles were presented in a manual, highlighting instructions for layout (see Figure 5.6) but also fitout, necessary kits, power, gas provision and ventilation. All patient beds were open plan with partitions at the head of the bed for servicing and the allocation of medical equipment. A typical ward arrangement saw nursing stations at either side of a long row of beds with a two-metre corridor between bed rows. Perpendicular to those corridors a clean route and a dirty route were arranged, separated only by distance, not by walls. With no actual partitions and all air exchanges centrally organised in the large halls, ventilation strategies relied on air flowing from clean to dirty areas. In effect, the clean and dirty separations were therefore less rigorously conceived than in the Chinese Wuhan COVID-hospitals.

Reflections by BDP Principal Ged Couser highlight the speed and scale of procurement, the collaborative practices in the process and the fact that this seemed like the right thing to do at the time, not knowing enough about COVID as a disease, or how harshly the healthcare system would actually be hit.[23] Systematic evaluations of the performance of the NHS Nightingale London were published by a team of medical practitioners having run the hospital. They reported that 54 patients in total were cared for and comparable outcomes to other NHS sites were confirmed, for instance regarding death rates, despite unforeseen challenges with the multi-faceted nature of COVID symptoms including multi-organ failure, which the Nightingales as critical emergency-care models were not well enough equipped to deal with effectively.[24]

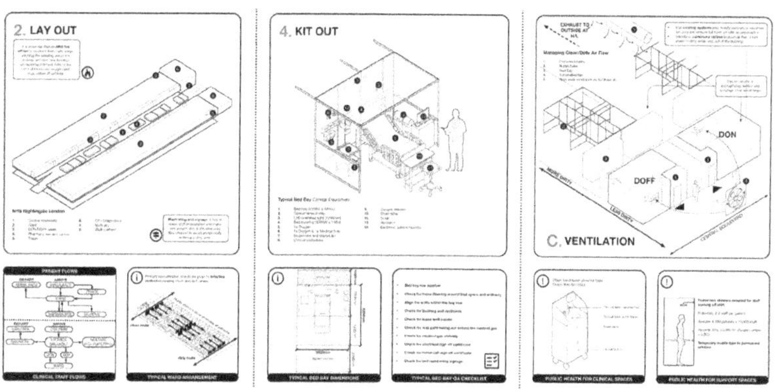

5.6 Layout, kit out and ventilation principles from the NHS Nightingale manual. Image courtesy of BDP.

In summary, the spatial and architectural strategies employed in the United Kingdom to manage the COVID pandemic included local decision making, small changes on the ground undertaken in relative separation in each hospital and the provision of emergency critical care in the NHS Nightingale structures. The NHS Nightingale hospitals, however, were used only for a very small number of patients, and therefore had little influence on the overall disease management.

Design as a response to (changing) priorities

It might seem commonplace to state this explicitly, but how hospitals are structured both organisationally and spatially, and therefore in turn how architects might make choices in their healthcare design projects, can be seen as a direct response to priorities.

Design responses to the pandemic mirrored underlying assumptions of what COVID-appropriate care looks like. In China, for instance, the experience with earlier coronaviruses and other infectious diseases created a strong blueprint and common understanding for necessary spatial elements such as triaging or the strict separation of movement flows in the interest of absolute infection prevention and control. Closed patient rooms were therefore a natural response. In the same vein, the strong Nightingale open-plan tradition in the United Kingdom meant that ideas of effective care automatically included the view of nurses in maintaining patient oversight, which led to an accommodation of patients in larger open-plan bays or halls.

What is more, the Huoshenshan emergency hospital had a single focused priority: preventing COVID deaths in both patients and healthcare workers. The system functioned so well, exactly because it worked alongside existing hospitals covering ongoing standard care as well as shelter hospitals caring for those with a mild course of disease. This is very different from the United Kingdom, where existing hospitals were adapted in the main and had to cover all of the above functions simultaneously (emergency intensive care, ongoing care and looking after patients with mild symptoms) and were thus torn. A combination of specialised building types providing nuanced and highly tailored care seemed the more successful strategy.[25]

There is another point worth making in our attempts to learn from COVID for hospital design in general, and that is how every design choice has an impact on the levels of social solidarities enfolding. The Huoshenshan model delivers an almost non-existent sociality. In fact, the experience of healthcare workers[26] seems to be one of gruelling isolation.

As a temporary approach and in the light of the primacy of avoiding nosocomial infection of healthcare workers, this appears like a price worth paying. On the contrary, a strong programme of social exchange was built into the design of the Fangcang shelter hospitals, showing how important solidarities and shared activities are for recovery. What can be learned here is possibly this: solidarities among people, among healthcare workers, between hospital staff and patients, between hospital staff and family are a crucial element of care. What has often been taken for granted, has suddenly been at stake due to the impact of the pandemic.

Solidarities and co-presence as a crucial need

Those of us living through COVID in countries with less of a grip on containing the spread of the virus will intuitively know what it means to be deprived of copresence. With repeated lockdowns, stay-at-home orders and contact limitations in place, our COVID-stricken lives have shrunk considerably, both in terms of everyday geographic reach and the diversity of people we meet, since we are reduced to spaces of the interior, as architectural historian Annmarie Adams eloquently argued.[27] Contacts have become diminished to the closest of close ties – family, good friends, direct work colleagues – and often maintained via online tools. With this polarisation of spatial and social experiences, casual friendly encounters with those not quite called friends – the barista normally making your coffee, the co-worker from a different department, the other football fans in the pub – disappear, as argued in an astute article in *The Atlantic*.[28] Different intensities of solidarity, both strong and weak ties[29] and everything in-between, are so important to humans, as they relate directly to how we have evolved as a species[30] and have continued to thrive, not as individuals and not just in small kinship related groups, but as 'social animals' in larger congregations and societies, connected to others in an intricate tangle of relations.[31]

In the same way in which solidarities matter in everyday life and similarly to how encounter structures have been uprooted by COVID, hospital life has changed dramatically. This transformation can be described by referring back to early space syntax theorising in Hillier and Hanson's *The Social Logic of Space*.[32] In this seminal book, the authors argue that human relations are grounded in two different principles: spatial solidarities arising from physical closeness, and so-called 'transpatial'[33] solidarities emerging from conceptual closeness. In the most immediate sense, two people occupying the same physical space, able to perceive one another, can be considered co-present[34] and thus engaged in a spatial form of solidarity, since awareness of other people forms the raw material of what Hillier calls 'virtual community'.[35] In contrast, physical distance can be overcome if people have things in common and therefore a motivation to invest in a relationship. Applying those two dimensions to hospitals – spatial and transpatial – we can easily see that communities are structured both around spatial co-presence and working together (communities of interest, e.g., all healthcare workers populating a ward and looking after the welfare of patients), but also around transpatial professions and roles (communities of practice, e.g., all nurses, porters or cleaners following particular codes of conduct). In times of COVID, I would argue, hospitals were forced to tone down spatial solidarities and have thus become more transpatially organised. For instance, visitors were no longer allowed on wards by default and were invited only under special circumstances, so that the majority of exchange between patients and family had to take place via videocalls. It has already been argued that the segregating layout of Chinese emergency makeshift hospitals took away opportunities for healthcare worker solidarities for the sake of infection control. Likewise, staff fully geared up with several layers of PPE can often no longer recognise their own colleagues, as faces and bodies are hidden. With administrative staff and hospital planners working from home where possible, it is easy to see how spatial solidarities were reduced.

Yet another relationship between spatial and transpatial solidarities can be brought to bear in this discussion and that is the differentiation between systems of correspondence or non-correspondence, again following Hillier and Hanson's argument. A correspondent system, one in which spatial and transpatial solidarities correspond to a high degree, can be described as locally strong, exclusive and hierarchical with pronounced boundaries. Correspondent systems often form segregated islands, within which people are both brought together by spatial proximity but also by conceptual closeness yet reaching across those silos can become difficult. In contrast, a non-correspondent system allows spatial proximity to overcome conceptual difference or vice versa, leading to a system characterised by openness, equality, inclusivity and global strength.[36] Under normal operations, hospitals could be argued to oscillate between correspondence and non-correspondence, for example a tearoom exclusively used by nurses presents a place of correspondence. In the same vein, doctors, cleaners or porters might have their own break rooms or spaces to congregate. These spaces nurture within group solidarities and allow strong ties to form. Other places in the hospital, notably corridors, are a shared space for non-correspondence. Different groups come together, thus allowing weaker ties to emerge and for the whole system to be pulled together. The nursing station in a ward, despite suggesting a gathering of nurses is also often a place where different groups of professionals congregate.[37] In the same way that COVID diminished spatial relations in hospitals, solidarities were also shifted to a higher degree of correspondence. Corridors for example became potential vectors of infection and were avoided where possible. Congregations between different groups of people were reduced to a bare minimum. And maybe most painfully, spaces much needed for comfort and respite for staff to cope with increased pressures at work (e.g, tearooms) were traced as a root cause of nosocomial infections in staff.[38]

One of the many dilemmas of the pandemic is therefore that it forces us apart in times when we dearly require human connection; human connections are best made in physical space, yet that physical space becomes dangerous:

> Of all COVID's cruelties, surely the greatest is this? That it cleaves us from each other at precisely those times when we need human contact the most. That it spreads through speech and touch – the very means through which we share our love, tenderness and basic humanity. That it transforms us unwittingly into vectors of fatality. And that those we love most – and with whom we are most intimate – are the ones we endanger above all others.[39]

In summary, solidarities in hospitals can be expressed under distinct conditions of correspondence or non-correspondence, thus bringing together single or different groups of people. Solidarities help to humanise healthcare by supporting team efforts, but also giving people access to comfort and empathy, as well as sharing the burden of responsibilities. All these functions are enabled by physical space providing co-presence, but with pandemic-related precautions and changes in routines, spatial closeness as well as non-correspondence have become compromised and reduced. For this very reason and reflecting on the deprivations caused by COVID, Klinenberg calls for gathering places for people to come together across all divides to strengthen solidarities for the post-pandemic future we need to rebuild.[40]

Designing the future hospital: user-centric healthcare design

It is finally time to raise the question of how the insights generated from the research presented in this chapter and the wider book can be turned into a set of coherent design principles. This involves bridging between academic circles and design practitioners. Much has been said about this topic over the decades – from the reflective practitioner[41] to reconciling intellect and intuition[42]; from evidence-based design[43] to pre and post studies[44] and randomised controlled trials[45] featuring hospital design.

A recent reflection by Michael Batty on the relationship between science and design brings the challenge to the point:

> Science and design require different perspectives on the world, and although in theory, most believe that good science and good design go hand-in-hand, the differences in viewpoint are significant enough to make the question continually challenging. It is almost a rite of passage to argue that science and design both require intuition and discipline ... but to ensure that [meeting goals] is possible, it remains forever problematic.[46]

We can therefore accept that translating scientific evidence and metrics back to the level of decision making of designers is not straightforward. Bafna and Zook have already outlined in Chapter 4 of this book how even explicit design guidelines on corridors can result in layouts that are contrary to the desired outcomes of easy wayfinding, if the space – designed with the best of intentions – is evaluated after completion.

This could be thought of as a problem of unintended consequences, defined by sociologist Robert Merton as a series of factors limiting the correct anticipation of consequences of action. Merton identified five such factors, including simpler explanations such as ignorance (1) and error (2), but also misjudgements due to an immediacy of diverging interests (3) or fundamental values (4), or in fact that consequences do not occur because of an interference from public predictions (5) (i.e., an outcome is anticipated and announced but does not happen since people actively changed the course of events in between).[47]

If we apply this scheme to healthcare and hospital design, factors 4 and 5 are arguably less relevant in design practice. On the contrary, ignorance and error might account for a reasonable number of unintended consequences. This is not meant in an antagonistic way – surely errors of this kind do not occur out of bad will, but due to the nature of design as a 'wicked problem', one that evades easy solving through scientific rationales.[48] We should also keep in mind how young and unestablished evidence-based design still is as a discipline.[49] As a result, errors may come into play through uncertainty, simply not knowing or wishful thinking. In addition, as a field we do not test our assumptions regularly enough. Every building could be conceived as an untested hypothesis, since designers and clients implement ideas of how an organisation might behave by means of spatial design. This is fine by itself, but the issue is that we too rarely test in a thorough way whether predictions that the building makes were actually realised. The third factor that Merton identified – an immediacy of interests – could also come into play, as design is project-based and aimed at solving problems of a particular client. Once a problem is solved and a project is delivered, teams are mostly disbanded and move on. Successful learning, for example through post-occupancy evaluations (or 'POE') often remains underfunded and undervalued,[50] but can still play a crucial part if implemented (e.g., as described by Nanda in her essay in this book).

Apart from unintended consequences, research in this domain of analytical design is predominantly looking backwards, at completed buildings and how they performed post hoc. While we can build on a rich tradition of research investigating the syntactical properties of viewsheds, strategic visibility and network structures in existing floorplans of hospitals, we hardly ever conduct research on how to design for various spatial outcomes. Exceptions to this norm are few and far between. Pachilova and Sailer offer a view in Chapter 3 of how particular and very concrete design decisions (e.g., to widen a corridor) result in larger strategic viewsheds, thus leading to a higher Spaces for Communication Index, which in turn was associated with better care quality. Another example outside of the hospital realm comes from the interdisciplinary work of Ruth Conroy Dalton in supporting game designers in the creation of different levels of difficulty of navigability in the game SeaHeroQuest, which was then used to study orientation skills of healthy populations for the benefit of dementia research. The task that Conroy Dalton faced was how to design environments with a pre-defined controllable difficulty in wayfinding.[51] The space syntax metric of intelligibility could be employed, as it was associated with ease of wayfinding, as evidenced in retrospective studies. However, turning retrospective insights on intelligibility levels of existing plans into prospective design principles was still a tricky process and something that is not often done in research.

Intelligibility as a composite metric[52] provides another pointer to further difficulties in translating research into practice. Scientists have developed increasingly complex ways of measuring spatial properties in floorplans in relation to behavioural outcomes. An example from hospital design is Lu's metric of targeted visibility, which describes not what someone can see from anywhere in the plan, but how visible certain targets (in this case patient beds) are. Lu found that targeted visibility predicted the location of nurses in a hospital ward better than generic visibility measures.[53] Another example from a different domain, office environments, shows how the locations of moving and interacting people in workplaces can be predicted well with aggregate metrics, for example floor by floor,[54] yet these aggregations are meaningless to designers, because no designer ever thinks about aggregate qualities of a building floor when making design decisions. While certainly of interest from a research point of view, complex, composite or aggregate metrics give little guidance to designers regarding how to design. The discrepancy between what designers design (e.g., walls, sizes of rooms, openings) and what scientists typically measure, exacerbates the problem of bridging academic research and practice.

It is argued here that building these bridges is not simply a matter of practitioners overcoming barriers, as a recent journal paper suggested,[55] but arguably at the same time we need to reflect on our contribution coming out of academic research as scientists, not just in terms of communication and accessible science, but also regarding the applicability of metrics.

With both practitioners and scientists doing their best to make research actionable, we can begin to address what to design for. At its most basic level, hospitals, it could be argued, battle with competing priorities. The example of China's COVID response shows how new, specialised building types were invented to cope with rapidly changing demands, thus intelligently evading the issue of competing priorities. Where this did not happen (e.g., in the United Kingdom), hospitals struggled with the need to balance different sets of priorities within a single building type – keeping staff safe, caring for unprecedented numbers of intensive care patients simultaneously, staying in touch with family and friends of patients while simultaneously trying to retain standard care procedures that could not be completely cancelled or postponed for extended periods. Arguably, COVID has taken these dilemmas to the extremes. Still, competing and at times contradictory priorities have been part of healthcare design for the longest time.

Engaging with practitioners therefore forces scientists out of the rabbit warrens (or ivory towers, whichever metaphor you prefer), that is, out of their deep subject knowledge, to appreciate the bigger picture.

Possibly, this is one of the contributions of this book, juxtaposing original research with practitioners' responses throughout.

So, let us ask: How should we design hospital corridors? With a focus on the whole hospital as a readable system, as highlighted by Bafna and Zook, thus bringing visitors, their cognitive capabilities and orientation issues as irregular building users to the forefront? Or with a focus on the movement of staff and stuff, thus supporting regular and routinised building functions? Where do the public-corridor system for patients and the ward-corridor system inhabited by professionals meet and how can inpatient unit corridors make visitors feel welcome, but at the same time also play a role for inter-professional communication, where boundaries between people in different roles are relaxed, as argued by Pachilova and Sailer?

How should beds be arranged? In single-patient rooms, as represented in the research of Ossmann or the contributions of Tingwald and Nanda, common in the United States? Or in open-plan wards, featured predominantly in the research of Pachilova and Sailer and representative of the UK tradition?

Who should be given priority as a user group when we design? The preferences of nurses, as signalled in the work of Ossmann? Or family and patients as a separate user group, as maintained by Tingwald? Or different user personas as proposed by Giannasca?

This brings us to our last section, reflecting on the question regarding which of the many users a design should serve first and foremost, and how user needs can be balanced.

Balancing user needs: which user anyway?

Reflecting on user needs, and who it is that is considered a 'user', bring to light once more how complex the hospital is as a building type. In their early work, Hillier and Hanson[56] distinguished inhabitants, those whose social knowledge is inscribed into the building and therefore control it, and visitors, who only have temporary rights to the building. It is easy to recognise these two categories as doctors and patients, and this is also how the authors proceed in their discussion. According to Hillier and Hanson the complexity of the hospital arises from the different types of interface that the modern hospital provides – how and where doctors meet patients, and who is in control of which spaces. Access to the hospital at large is only weakly controlled. Once inside, visitors can roam freely at first, also meeting each other. Outpatients accessing particular clinics move towards doctors, who are accommodated deep in the building, whereas inpatients in wards are in the deepest parts with the doctors circulating. Thus, Hillier and Hanson summarise:

> The hospital is, in effect, a nexus of potentially conflicting and contradictory socio-spatial forces, each in itself well defined but each as likely as another to gain a temporary ascendency in the evolution of designs. The hospital is characterised not so much by a single genotype, but by a genotypical conflict, perhaps one whose resolution is largely illusory.[57]

If we add to that analysis the problem that of course not all inhabitants (i.e., hospital staff) are doctors (but also nurses, porters, cleaners, anaesthetists, physiotherapists and medical students, to name just a few), and not all visitors are patients (but also family and friends), and recognise that each group comes with its own set of purposes, preferences and requirements, therefore both inhabitant and visitor categories multiply with differential levels of access, mobility, power and control. Mapping those patterns to building structures could of course be undertaken as a research project but would not bring us any closer to the question of resolving what Hillier and Hanson called 'largely illusory'.

There is yet another angle that can be usefully added to the discussion of which users should be considered. The majority of the literature on evidence-based or user-centric design conceptualises the user through individual-level responses – for example, how someone reacts to daylight, views of nature or the display of art. All these responses are of course important and should not be disregarded. It is also easy to explain how we have arrived at that point with a close involvement of environmental psychologists at the heart of the evidence-based design movement, as evident in the leading role of international associations such as the Environmental Design Research Association and the International Association of People-Environment Studies.[58] However, there is also a collective user to consider rather than just focusing on the hospital as an aggregation of individuals, each with their own preferences and predicaments.

This shift in perspective is fundamental since it conceptualises users not just as demographic groups but takes the interactions and relationships between those groups into account in a systematic way. A parallel can be drawn to the shift in the perception of public health that COVID has brought about, as argued earlier in this chapter. Where public health evaluations were traditionally applied to aggregated groups of people based on demographic characteristics, it is high time we rethink health as an interconnected system of opportunities and risks, not just deriving from someone's individual profile but also from their exposure to and relations with others.

Examples of this shift in perspective can be seen all throughout this book. Bafna and Zook bring individual cognitive processes of users together with the impact that the presence of others has, for example, in considering perceived usage conflicts in corridors. Reviews of buildings showcased profoundly how use is not a singular process in the absence of others but rather a layering of experiences and processes going on simultaneously (a safety officer questioning a visitor taking a selfie, a visitor irritated about a staff barbecue); or following Bafna and Zook, corridor systems are social in ways that convey institutional character and expectations. As such, corridors are considered as 'networked behaviour settings'.

Ossmann takes up the idea of the relational user by systematically considering nurses in direct relation to patients. With an interest in surveillance as a construct, the developed metric of concurrent visibility expresses not just the visual field from the head of a patient bed as a preferred location for nurses, but also the quality of spaces and visibility from within it, thereby taking into account how easily nurses can interact with each other while keeping an eye on the patient. Thus, Ossmann conceptualises users through the patient-nurse and the nurse-to-nurse relationship at the same time.

Pachilova and Sailer interpret relational users by including the whole team of healthcare workers on wards, as any person might become a crucial communication partner to a nurse on their everyday paths. The developed Spaces for Communication Index therefore operationalises aggregate viewshed sizes as nurses move through the ward as a proxy for communication opportunities. This approach is possibly taking the concept of a relational user furthest by applying a truly collective lens and considering a 'herd' user.

Therefore, in this book we show how we can rise to the challenge laid out by Hillier and Hanson decades ago and investigate the spatial conditions underlying multiple and complex interfaces, while simultaneously shifting from an individual user-centric approach to a collective and relational viewpoint.

A last point needs making, and that is how to finally balance competing user requirements. Before we can balance, however, user needs must be articulated and understood. Giannasca offers an approach in his response essay based on personas, as does Tingwald in highlighting how different groups might assess a potential building differently. Nanda proposes a layered design diagnostics approach, bringing different viewpoints together. By making perspectives explicit, design research, whether in academia or in practice, allows issues to surface. Discussing them openly within and across the design team, including the different stakeholder groups is a first step towards achieving balance. We also need to acknowledge that resolution of conflicting interests might differ from case to case. This localised stance has the advantage of avoiding unsolvable ethical dilemmas, as described in the classic trolley problem, for example. Design decisions of this nature can never be automated, as they require human empathy. Where an AI[59] requires generic, hard and fast rules of who to prioritise, judgements can be made one case at a time and become grounded in local preferences, situations and cultures.[60]

Therefore, the act of balancing competing priorities can be understood as a practice, where the process matters and not just the outcome. Practices have an everyday nature and are constituted by recursive human actions.[61] If we continuously work on putting users at the heart of hospital design, the following questions can accompany us: How can we better understand the (unintended) consequences of design decisions? How can we appreciate collective, overlapping and contradictory uses? How can we calibrate or balance competing requirements? Both academia and design practice have answers to contribute to this debate. The social and relational stance I have sketched here, I would argue, can make hospital architecture of the twenty-first century more likely to succeed, whether or not we are indeed facing a new 'age of pandemics'.

Notes

1 It is always much easier to judge events and actions in hindsight, which is brilliantly summarised in Duncan J. Watts, *Everything is Obvious: Once You Know the Answer* (Crown Business, 2011).

2 Clarke, Rachel, *Breath Taking: Inside the NHS in a Time of Pandemic* (London: Little, Brown, 2021). The quote is on page 108, where Clarke explains the differences between the COVID-19 emergency and other major incidents that the NHS has planned for.

3 Pre-pandemic trends in other domains such as office life or education were accelerated as well, for instance, the rising acceptance of working from home and flexible working, or the increase in online seminars and flipped classroom teaching.

4 In fact, this perspective is not entirely new and has not appeared out of thin air just because of COVID. Social network research has long argued that relationships matter and that our (health) behaviours do not stem only from individual-level attributes (sex, age, educational level, income, ethnicity, etc.), but also from the influence of our friends, peers and closest ties. For an overview of social networks and health, see Thomas W. Valente, *Social Networks and Health: Models, Methods, and Applications* (Oxford and New York: Oxford University Press, 2010).

5 Detailed examples of all four strategies are presented on a website, collected as part of a research project initiated by the European Health Property Network EuHPN and hosted by

Ramboll, a global engineering, architecture and consultancy company founded in Denmark. See Ramboll, 'Pandemic resilience: space adaptation' (Copenhagen: Ramboll, 2021) (accessed 1 March 2021), https://c.ramboll.com/pandemic-resilience-space.

6 This and all following references to the timeline of events unfolding in China were taken from the overview of the World Health Organization, https://www.who.int/news/item/29-06-2020-covidtimeline (accessed 3 March 2021), as well as a detailed chronology of events provided by the initiative Think Global Health; see 'Updated: timeline of the coronavirus' (Think Global Health, 2021), https://www.thinkglobalhealth.org/article/updated-timeline-coronavirus (accessed 3 March 2021).

7 Figures for the cumulative number of deaths for China and the United Kingdom were taken from the Coronavirus Resource Center run by the Johns Hopkins University of Medicine, https://coronavirus.jhu.edu/map.html (accessed 3 March 2021).

8 This *Lancet* article gives a good overview of China's response: Talha Burki, 'China's successful control of COVID-19', *The Lancet Infectious Diseases*, 20, no. 11 (8 October 2020), https://doi.org/10.1016/S1473-3099(20)30800-8. In addition, a summary by the international volunteer coalition End Coronavirus, initiated by the New England Complex Systems Institute (NECSI) evaluates different strategies in principle: 'Unsuccessful versus successful Covid strategies' (New England Complex Systems Institute, 2020), https://www.endcoronavirus.org/papers/covid-strategies (accessed 13 December 2020).

9 Zhou Lihua *et al.*, 'Workers race against time to build "high-speed" hospitals', *China Daily Global Edition* (Hong Kong, 1 February 2020), https://www.chinadailyhk.com/article/119829.

10 Burki, 'China's successful control of COVID-19'.

11 Simiao Chen *et al.*, 'Fangcang shelter hospitals: a novel concept for responding to public health emergencies', *The Lancet*, 395, no. 10232 (2020), https://doi.org/10.1016/S0140-6736(20)30744-3.

12 Jie Li *et al.*, '"Re-socialisation" in isolated spaces: a case study on the social organisation of Fangcang shelter hospital patients under extreme spatial conditions', *Indoor and Built Environment*, online first (2020), https://doi.org/10.1177/1420326x20973745, https://journals.sagepub.com/doi/abs/10.1177/1420326X20973745.

13 It is now assumed that COVID circulated in the United Kingdom much earlier, yet 1 February is still the accepted date for a first confirmed case. Detailed dates and events of how COVID evolved in the United Kingdom will be taken from a timeline published by the British weekly news magazine *The Week*; see 'The UK's coronavirus pandemic timeline', *The Week* (2021), https://www.theweek.co.uk/107044/uk-coronavirus-timeline (accessed 1 March 2021).

14 At the time of writing, the United Kingdom ranked fifth in death numbers, overtaken only by the United States (540,000+), Brazil (300,000+), Mexico (200,000+) and India (160,000+) according to the Johns Hopkins dashboard – all in countries with much larger populations, at least twice the size of the United Kingdom (in the case of Mexico), or in a different order of magnitude (in the case of India). Only much smaller countries, such as the Czech Republic, Belgium and Slovenia had higher death rates per inhabitants; see https://www.statista.com/statistics/1104709/coronavirus-deaths-worldwide-per-million-inhabitants/ (accessed 3 March 2021).

15 The ambivalence of communication is perhaps most aptly displayed in a press conference on 3 March 2020, when Prime Minister Boris Johnson told he had visited a hospital with COVID patients and continued shaking hands with everyone, against advice by the government's Scientific Advisory Group for Emergencies (known as 'SAGE') to limit hand shaking and other forms of direct contact, issued on the same day. The slow UK response is also eloquently critiqued in Michael Rosen, *Many Different Kinds of Love: A Story of Life, Death and the NHS* (London: Ebury Publishing, 2021).

16 BBC World Service, *Part One: The Coronavirus Front Line*, episode 1 of 8, podcast audio (2020), https://www.bbc.co.uk/programmes/w3ct0s1c.

17 BBC World Service, *Bradford Royal Infirmary: Another week in the ward fighting against Covid-19: The Coronavirus Front Line*, episode 3 of 8, podcast audio (2020), https://www.bbc.co.uk/programmes/w3ct0s1f.

18 BBC World Service, *The Coronavirus Front Line*, episode 6 of 8, podcast audio (2020), https://www.bbc.co.uk/programmes/w3ct0t4j.

19 Sarah Boseley, 'Key London hospital preparing for Covid-only care as cases surge', *Guardian* (London and Manchester, 2020), https://www.theguardian.com/world/2020/dec/31/london-hospital-uclh-warns-on-track-become-covid-only.

20 Clarke, *Breath Taking: Inside the NHS in a Time of Pandemic*.

21 It is estimated that at least 850 healthcare workers in the United Kingdom died of COVID; see David Berger, 'Up the line to death: Covid-19 has revealed a mortal betrayal of the world's healthcare workers', *The BMJ Opinion*, *British Medical Journal* (29 January 2021), https://blogs.bmj.com/bmj/2021/01/29/up-the-line-to-death-covid-19-has-revealed-a-mortal-betrayal-of-the-worlds-healthcare-workers/.

22 A brief description of the project can be found on the website of the lead architect BDP: https://www.bdp.com/en/projects/m-o/nhs-nightingale-hospital/ (accessed 9 February 2021).

23 These insights are based on a private telephone conversation on 12 February 2021 with Ged Couser, BDP Principal and lead architect of the NHS Nightingale hospitals.

24 Alastair G. Proudfoot *et al.*, 'Rapid establishment of a COVID-19 critical care unit in a convention centre: the Nightingale Hospital London experience', *Intensive Care Medicine* (2021), https://doi.org/10.1007/s00134-020-06334-6.

25 The idea of specialised new building types in healthcare architecture is also discussed in Chapter 1 of this book by Zook.

26 Very little has emerged on what it was like to work in one of those hospitals. The documentary CoroNation by Chinese provocateur Ai Weiwei gives some clues. A review of the documentary summarises: 'There's an amazing shot near the film's beginning in which the camera follows one medical worker through a windowless corridor. Wisely, there's nary a cut – the shot goes on and on and on for several minutes as the worker winds past various windowless rooms. We glimpse others along the way – some are putting on PPE, others seem to be performing medical tests – but the worker curiously ignores them. The corridor is dark and seemingly infinite, but somehow, the subject knows where to go.' See Alex Greenberger, 'Ai Weiwei's suprise-release Wuhan film is a gripping document of the coronavirus pandemic's beginning', *ARThews* (24 August 2020), https://www.artnews.com/art-news/news/ai-weiwei-coronation-film-review-1202697762/.

27 Annmarie Adams, 'This is where we live', *Parlour: Women, Equity, Architecture* (16 November 2020), https://archiparlour.org/this-is-where-we-live/.equity.

28 Amanda Mull, 'The pandemic has erased entire categories of friendship', *The Atlantic* (27 January 2021), https://www.theatlantic.com/health/archive/2021/01/pandemic-goodbye-casual-friends/617839/.

29 The importance of not just our strongest ties, our inner circle of close family and friends was most prominently shown by the work of sociologist Mark Granovetter in his seminal paper 'The strength of weak ties'. In it he argues that strong ties (i.e., those people we see regularly and often) do not give us access to new information or new knowledge, whereas weaker ties with loose friends and acquaintances (i.e., those we see less often) can bring real advantages, for example in job searches. For the full argument, see Mark S. Granovetter, 'The strength of weak ties', *The American Journal of Sociology*, 78, no. 6 (1973).

30 Anthropologist Robin Dunbar has suggested the number 150 as a recurring size of human social networks, from hunter-gatherer societies to military structures, linking group sizes to evolution, the size of the human neocortex and human social cognitive capacity; see Russell A. Hill and Robin I. M. Dunbar, 'Social network size in humans', *Human Nature*, 14, no. 1 (2003), http://dx.doi.org/10.1007/s12110-003-1016-y; Robin I. M. Dunbar, 'The social brain: mind, language, and society in evolutionary perspective', *Annual Review of Anthropology*, 32 (2003), http://www.jstor.org/stable/25064825.

31 How this relates to the division of labour as a social function maintaining society is discussed more in depth in Pachilova and Sailer in Chapter 3 of this book.

32 Bill Hillier and Julienne Hanson, *The Social Logic of Space* (Cambridge: Cambridge University Press, 1984).

33 Hillier's and Hanson's rationale in naming the second category as 'transpatial' is not explicitly spelled out but can be easily explained as that which is non-spatial or, more accurately, as the kind of relations that can traverse spatial distances (i.e., going beyond space). Authors from other domains might call these relations simply 'social'. In the field of social network analysis, authors would refer to 'homophily', or the principle that 'birds of a feather flock together'; J. Miller McPherson, Lynn Smith-Lovin and James M. Cook, 'Birds of a feather: homophily in social networks', *Annual Review of Sociology*, 27, no. 1 (2001), https://doi.org/doi:10.1146/annurev.soc.27.1.415; http://arjournals.annualreviews.org/doi/abs/10.1146/annurev.soc.27.1.415.

34 A useful differentiation and definition of co-presence is offered by Netto *et al.* as 'bodies positioned within a field where we can perceive the presence of another person', which is distinguished from both encounter (i.e., 'co-present within a distance where interaction

becomes possible') and interaction (i.e., 'engaging in communicative exchange'). See Vicinius M. Netto *et al.*, 'A temporal geography of encounters', *Cybergeo: European Journal of Geography, Space, Society, Territory* (5 February 2018), https://doi.org/10.4000/cybergeo.28985.

35 Co-presence, Hillier argues, is not the same as community, but is its raw material, since social opportunities can become activated, if necessary. Interestingly, Netto *et al.* maintain that encounter is the raw material of social life, in contrast to Hillier, who argues for co-presence as foundation. See Bill Hillier, *Space is the Machine: A Configurational Theory of Architecture* (Cambridge: Cambridge University Press, 1996), https://discovery.ucl.ac.uk/id/eprint/3881/1/SITM.pdf.

36 For a description of correspondence and non-correspondence Hillier and Hanson use academics as an example, who come together at conferences temporarily (correspondence), but typically topic experts are spread around the globe (non-correspondence). The overall strength that a non-correspondent system provides has also been called a 'social insurance policy' by Peponis and linked to innovative capacity by Sailer and Thomas. See John Peponis, 'Interacting questions and descriptions: how do they look from here?' (paper presented at the 3rd International Space Syntax Symposium, Atlanta GA, 2001); Kerstin Sailer and Matt Thomas, 'Correspondence and non-correspondence: using office accommodation to calculate an organization's propensity for new ideas' (paper presented at the 12th International Space Syntax Symposium, Beijing, China, 2019).

37 Rosica Pachilova, 'Exploring quality of care in hospital wards: the effect of spatial layout, staff work activities and communication patterns' (PhD, UCL, 2020), https://discovery.ucl.ac.uk/id/eprint/10093866/.

38 A small-scale study in an Australian hospital reported a cluster of staff infections that could be traced back to an infected and not yet diagnosed member of staff spending time with colleagues in a staff tearoom, who also subsequently became infected with COVID-19. See Claire L. Gordon *et al.*, 'Staff to staff transmission as a driver of healthcare worker infections with COVID-19', *medRxiv* (2020), https://doi.org/https://doi.org/10.1101/2020.12.25.20248824.

39 A reflection in February 2021 offered by UK doctor Rachel Clarke in her newspaper article '"I've been called Satan": Dr Rachel Clarke on facing abuse in the Covid crisis' (6 February 2021), https://www.theguardian.com/books/2021/feb/06/ive-been-called-satan-dr-rachel-clarke-on-facing-abuse-in-the-covid-crisis (accessed 8 February 2021).

40 Eric Klinenberg, 'Rebuilding solidarity in a broken world', *Public Books* (27 November 2020), https://www.publicbooks.org/rebuilding-solidarity-in-a-broken-world/.

41 Donald A. Schön, *The Reflective Practitioner: How Professionals Think in Action* (Aldershot: Ashgate Publishing Limited, 1991).

42 Julienne Hanson, 'Morphology and design: reconciling intellect, intuition and ethics in the reflective practice of architecture' (paper presented at the 3rd International Space Syntax Symposium, Atlanta GA, 2001).

43 Roger Ulrich *et al.*, *The Role of the Physical Environment in the Hospital of the 21st Century: A Once-in-a-Lifetime Opportunity* (Concord CA: The Center for Health Design, 2005), http://www.healthdesign.org/research/reports/pdfs/role_physical_env.pdf.

44 Kerstin Sailer *et al.*, 'Pre and post occupancy evaluations in workplace environments', *The Journal of Space Syntax*, 1, no. 1 (2010).

45 Diane P. Martin *et al.*, 'Randomized trial of a patient-centered hospital unit', *Patient Education and Counselling*, 34, no. 2 (June 1998), https://doi.org/10.1016/s0738-3991(97)00089-x.

46 Michael Batty, 'Science and design in the age of COVID-19', *Environment and Planning B: Urban Analytics and City Science*, 48, no. 1 (2021), 3, https://journals.sagepub.com/doi/abs/10.1177/2399808321989131.

47 Robert K. Merton, 'The unanticipated consequences of purposive social action', *American Sociological Review*, 1, no. 6 (1936), https://doi.org/10.2307/2084615.

48 Horst W. J. Rittel and Melvin M. Webber, 'Dilemmas in a general theory of planning', *Policy Sciences*, 4 (1973).

49 Science historian Thomas Kuhn reminds us that established sciences such as physics have had centuries to test and trial explanations about the universe and the natural world. Medicine is often considered to have become a science in the nineteenth century, whereas psychology rose to prominence at the beginning of the twentieth century. In contrast, the consideration of human factors in organisations and therefore in design – with notable exceptions – did not emerge until after World War Two. See Thomas S. Kuhn, *The Structure of Scientific Revolutions* (3rd edition) (Chicago IL: University of Chicago Press, 1996).

50 Kerstin Sailer, 'The "P" in POE: pre, post or permanent occupancy evaluation?', *brainybirdz blog* (9 March 2020), https://brainybirdz.net/2020/03/09/the-p-in-poe-pre-post-or-permanent-occupancy-evaluation/.

51 An overview of the role of architectural design in the SeaHeroQuest project is given by Ruth Conroy Dalton, 'Want to build better computer games? Call an architect', *The Conversation* (6 May 2016), https://theconversation.com/want-to-build-better-computer-games-call-an-architect-58912. The remainder of the points discussed here were taken from Conroy Dalton's keynote speech at the 11th Space Syntax Symposium in Lisbon in 2017, which has not been published to the best of my knowledge.

52 Intelligibility describes the correlation between local and global information or, in other words, how well I can infer my position in a global network from what I can see locally. For a full description, see Hillier, *Space is the Machine: A Configurational Theory of Architecture*. Also refer to John Peponis, Craig Zimring and Yoon Kyung Choi, 'Finding the building in wayfinding', *Environment and Behavior*, 22, no. 5 (1990), https://doi.org/10.1177/0013916590225001.

53 Yi Lu and Craig Zimring, 'Can intensive care staff see their patients? An improved visibility analysis methodology', *Environment and Behavior*, 44, no. 6 (2011), https://doi.org/10.1177/0013916511405314.

54 Petros Koutsolampros, 'Human behaviour in office environments: finding patterns of activity and spatial configuration in large workplace datasets' (PhD, UCL, 2021).

55 Fouad Jalal Mahmood, 'The role of evidence-based design in informing healthcare architects', *Journal of Facilities Management* (2021), https://doi.org/10.1108/JFM-09-2020-0062.

56 Hillier and Hanson, *The Social Logic of Space*.

57 Hillier and Hanson, *The Social Logic of Space*, 192–3.

58 Information about the Environmental Design Research Association and the International Association of People-Environment Studies can be found at: https://www.edra.org/default.aspx and https://iaps-association.org/ (accessed 11 March 2021).

59 A comprehensive discussion of ethical dilemmas, algorithmic biases and perverse incentives that present when choices have to be hard-coded, such as for driverless cars, is provided in Hazel Si Min Lim and Araz Taeihagh, 'Algorithmic decision-making in AVs: understanding ethical and technical concerns for smart cities', *Sustainability*, 11, no. 20 (2019), https://www.mdpi.com/2071-1050/11/20/5791.

60 A good example of how ward structures are perceived differently as a result of cultural influences is provided by Hui Cai and Craig Zimring, 'Cultural impacts on nursing unit design: a comparative study on Chinese nursing unit typologies and their U.S. counterparts using space syntax', *Environment and Planning B: Urban Analytics and City Science*, 46, no. 3 (2019), http://journals.sagepub.com/doi/abs/10.1177/2399808317715639.

61 Anthony Giddens, *The Constitution of Society: Outline of the Theory of Structuration* (Cambridge: Polity Press, 1984).

References

Adams, Annmarie, 'This is where we live', *Parlour: Women, Equity, Architecture* (16 November 2020), https://archiparlour.org/this-is-where-we-live/.

Batty, Michael, 'Science and design in the age of COVID-19', *Environment and Planning B: Urban Analytics and City Science*, 48, no. 1 (2021), 3–8, https://journals.sagepub.com/doi/abs/10.1177/2399808321989131.

BBC World Service, *Bradford Royal Infirmary: Another week in the ward fighting against Covid-19*, episode 3 of 8, podcast audio (The Documentary, 23 minutes, 2020), https://www.bbc.co.uk/programmes/w3ct0s1f.

BBC World Service, *The Coronavirus Front Line*, episode 6 of 8, podcast audio (The Documentary, 23 minutes, 2020), https://www.bbc.co.uk/programmes/w3ct0t4j.

BBC World Service, *Part One: The Coronavirus Front Line*, episode 1 of 8, podcast audio (The Documentary, 23 minutes, 2020), https://www.bbc.co.uk/programmes/w3ct0s1c.

Berger, David, 'Up the line to death: Covid-19 has revealed a mortal betrayal of the world's healthcare workers', *The BMJ Opinion*, *British Medical Journal* (29 January 2021), https://blogs.bmj.com/bmj/2021/01/29/up-the-line-to-death-covid-19-has-revealed-a-mortal-betrayal-of-the-worlds-healthcare-workers/.

Boseley, Sarah, 'Key London hospital preparing for Covid-only care as cases surge', *Guardian* (London and Manchester, 13 December 2020), https://www.theguardian.com/world/2020/dec/31/london-hospital-uclh-warns-on-track-become-covid-only.

Burki, Talha, 'China's successful control of COVID-19', *The Lancet Infectious Diseases*, 20, no. 11 (8 October 2020), 1240–1, https://doi.org/10.1016/S1473-3099(20)30800-8.

Cai, Hui, and Craig Zimring, 'Cultural impacts on nursing unit design: a comparative study on Chinese nursing unit typologies and their U.S. counterparts using space syntax', *Environment and Planning B: Urban Analytics and City Science*, 46, no. 3 (2019), 573–94, http://journals.sagepub.com/doi/abs/10.1177/2399808317715639.

Chen, Simiao, *et al.*, 'Fangcang shelter hospitals: a novel concept for responding to public health emergencies', *The Lancet*, 395, no. 10232 (2020), 1305–14, https://doi.org/10.1016/S0140-6736(20)30744-3.

Clarke, Rachel, *Breath Taking: Inside the NHS in a Time of Pandemic* (London: Little, Brown, 2021).

Clarke, Rachel, '"I've been called Satan": Dr Rachel Clarke on facing abuse in the Covid crisis', *Guardian* (London and Manchester, 6 February 2021), Books, https://www.theguardian.com/books/2021/feb/06/ive-been-called-satan-dr-rachel-clarke-on-facing-abuse-in-the-covid-crisis. (accessed 8 February 2021)

Conroy Dalton, Ruth, 'Want to build better computer games? Call an architect', *The Conversation* (6 May 2016), https://theconversation.com/want-to-build-better-computer-games-call-an-architect-58912.

Dunbar, Robin I. M., 'The social brain: mind, language, and society in evolutionary perspective', *Annual Review of Anthropology*, 32 (2003), 163–81, http://www.jstor.org/stable/25064825.

Environmental Design Research Association, https://www.edra.org/default.aspx (accessed 11 March 2021).

Giddens, Anthony, *The Constitution of Society: Outline of the Theory of Structuration* (Cambridge: Polity Press, 1984).

Gordon, Claire L., *et al.*, 'Staff to staff transmission as a driver of healthcare worker infections with COVID-19', *medRxiv* (2020), https://doi.org/10.1101/2020.12.25.20248824.

Granovetter, Mark S., 'The strength of weak ties', *The American Journal of Sociology*, 78, no. 6 (1973), 1360–80.

Greenberger, Alex, 'Ai Weiwei's suprise-release Wuhan film is a gripping document of the coronavirus pandemic's beginning', *ARTnews* (24 August 2020), https://www.artnews.com/art-news/news/ai-weiwei-coronation-film-review-1202697762/.

Hanson, Julienne, 'Morphology and design: reconciling intellect, intuition and ethics in the reflective practice of architecture' (paper presented at the 3rd International Space Syntax Symposium, Atlanta GA, 2001).

Hill, Russell A., and Robin I. M. Dunbar, 'Social network size in humans', *Human Nature*, 14, no. 1 (2003), 53–72, http://dx.doi.org/10.1007/s12110-003-1016-y.

Hillier, Bill, *Space is the Machine: A Configurational Theory of Architecture* (Cambridge: Cambridge University Press, 1996). https://discovery.ucl.ac.uk/id/eprint/3881/1/SITM.pdf.

Hillier, Bill, and Julienne Hanson, *The Social Logic of Space* (Cambridge: Cambridge University Press, 1984).
International Association of People-Environment Studies, https://iaps-association.org/ (accessed 11 March 2021).
Johns Hopkins University of Medicine Coronavirus Resource Center, 'COVID-19 Dashboard' (2021), https://coronavirus.jhu.edu/map.html (accessed 3 March 2021).
Klinenberg, Eric, 'Rebuilding solidarity in a broken world', *Public Books* (27 November 2020), https://www.publicbooks.org/rebuilding-solidarity-in-a-broken-world/.
Koutsolampros, Petros, 'Human behaviour in office environments: finding patterns of activity and spatial configuration in large workplace datasets' (PhD, UCL, 2021).
Kuhn, Thomas S., *The Structure of Scientific Revolutions* (3rd edition) (Chicago IL: University of Chicago Press, 1996).
Li, Jie, *et al.*, '"Re-socialisation" in isolated spaces: a case study on the social organisation of Fangcang shelter hospital patients under extreme spatial conditions', *Indoor and Built Environment*, online first (2020), https://doi.org/10.1177/1420326x20973745.
Lihua, Zhou, *et al.*, 'Workers race against time to build "high-speed" hospitals', *China Daily Global Edition* (Hong Kong) (1 February 2020), https://www.chinadailyhk.com/article/119829.
Lim, Hazel Si Min and Araz Taeihagh, 'Algorithmic decision-making in AVs: understanding ethical and technical concerns for smart cities', *Sustainability*, 11, no. 20 (2019), https://www.mdpi.com/2071-1050/11/20/5791.
Lu, Yi, and Craig Zimring, 'Can intensive care staff see their patients? An improved visibility analysis methodology', *Environment and Behavior*, 44, no. 6 (2011), 861–76, https://doi.org/10.1177/0013916511405314.
Mahmood, Fouad Jalal, 'The role of evidence-based design in informing healthcare architects', *Journal of Facilities Management*, online first (2021), https://doi.org/10.1108/JFM-09-2020-0062.
Martin, Diane P., *et al.*, 'Randomized trial of a patient-centered hospital unit', *Patient Education and Counselling*, 34, no. 2 (June 1998), 125–33, https://doi.org/10.1016/s0738-3991(97)00089-x.
McPherson, J. Miller, Lynn Smith-Lovin and James M. Cook, 'Birds of a feather: homophily in social networks', *Annual Review of Sociology*, 27, no. 1 (2001), 415–44, https://doi.org/10.1146/annurev.soc.27.1.415.
Merton, Robert K., 'The unanticipated consequences of purposive social action', *American Sociological Review*, 1, no. 6 (1936), 894–904, https://doi.org/10.2307/2084615.
Mull, Amanda, 'The pandemic has erased entire categories of friendship', *The Atlantic* (27 January 2021), https://www.theatlantic.com/health/archive/2021/01/pandemic-goodbye-casual-friends/617839/.
Netto, Vicinius M., *et al.*, 'A temporal geography of encounters', *Cybergeo: European Journal of Geography Space, Society, Territory* (5 February 2018), https://doi.org/10.4000/cybergeo.28985.
New England Complex Systems Institute (NECSI), 'Unsuccessful versus successful Covid strategies' (New England Complex Systems Institute, 2020), https://www.endcoronavirus.org/papers/covid-strategies (accessed 13 December 2020).
Pachilova, Rosica, 'Exploring quality of care in hospital wards: the effect of spatial layout, staff work activities and communication patterns' (PhD, UCL, 2020), https://discovery.ucl.ac.uk/id/eprint/10093866/.
Peponis, John, 'Interacting questions and descriptions: how do they look from here?' (paper presented at the 3rd International Space Syntax Symposium, Atlanta GA, 2001).
Peponis, John, Craig Zimring and Yoon Kyung Choi, 'Finding the building in wayfinding', *Environment and Behavior*, 22, no. 5 (1990), 555–90, https://doi.org/10.1177/0013916590225001.
Proudfoot, Alastair G., *et al.*, 'Rapid establishment of a COVID-19 critical care unit in a convention centre: the Nightingale Hospital London experience', *Intensive Care Medicine* (2021), https://doi.org/10.1007/s00134-020-06334-6.
Ramboll, 'Pandemic resilience: space adaptation' (Copenhagen: Ramboll, 2021), https://c.ramboll.com/pandemic-resilience-space. (accessed 1 March 2021)
Rittel, Horst W. J., and Melvin M. Webber, 'Dilemmas in a general theory of planning', *Policy Sciences*, 4 (1973), 155–69.

Rosen, Michael, *Many Different Kinds of Love: A Story of Life, Death and the NHS* (London: Ebury Publishing, 2021).

Sailer, Kerstin, 'The "P" in POE: pre, post or permanent occupancy evaluation?', *brainybirdz blog* (9 March 2020), https://brainybirdz.net/2020/03/09/the-p-in-poe-pre-post-or-permanent-occupancy-evaluation/.

Sailer, Kerstin, and Matt Thomas, 'Correspondence and non-correspondence: using office accommodation to calculate an organization's propensity for new ideas' (paper presented at the 12th International Space Syntax Symposium, Beijing, China, 2019).

Sailer, Kerstin, *et al.*, 'Pre and post occupancy evaluations in workplace environments', *The Journal of Space Syntax*, 1, no. 1 (2010), 199–213.

Schön, Donald A., *The Reflective Practitioner: How Professionals Think in Action* (Aldershot: Ashgate Publishing Limited, 1991).

Statista (2021), https://www.statista.com/statistics/1104709/coronavirus-deaths-worldwide-per-million-inhabitants/ (accessed 3 March 2021).

The Week, 'The UK's coronavirus pandemic timeline', *The Week* (2021), https://www.theweek.co.uk/107044/uk-coronavirus-timeline (accessed 1 March 2021).

Think Global Health, 'Updated: timeline of the coronavirus' (Think Global Health, 2021), https://www.thinkglobalhealth.org/article/updated-timeline-coronavirus.

Ulrich, Roger, *et al.*, *The Role of the Physical Environment in the Hospital of the 21st Century: A Once-in-a-Lifetime Opportunity* (Concord CA: The Center for Health Design, 2005), http://www.healthdesign.org/research/reports/pdfs/role_physical_env.pdf.

Valente, Thomas W., *Social Networks and Health: Models, Methods, and Applications* (Oxford and New York: Oxford University Press, 2010).

Watts, Duncan J., *Everything is Obvious: Once You Know the Answer* (Crown Business, 2011).

World Health Organization, 'Listings of WHO's response to COVID-19' (WHO 2020), https://www.who.int/news/item/29-06-2020-covidtimeline (accessed 3 March 2021).

Index

acute care, 25–8, 41–2, 69,
  see also intensive care
aesthetic, 8, 15–6,109–14
affordances, 29, 32–3, 36, 84, 85, 112
alcoves, 44–6
artwork, 114–115
awareness, 3, 93, 133, 141–2
  among coworkers, 40, 55, 66
  as part of surveillance, 25–6, 32–34

backstage, 67–68, 79
bedside, 25, 27–8
  care at, 39, 43–4, 69, 81, 84
behaviour settings, 6–8, 13–14, 109, 115, 149
Benedikt, Michael, 29–32
building codes, 13, 43–4

charting, 21, 28, 43–6
cognition, 2, 5, 97, 115, 131
cognitive map, 97, 100–2, 106, 116,
  see also hippocampal map
cohorting, 41
collaboration, 55, 58, 66–8, 74–5, 82
communication,
  care team communication, 25–6, 66–8, 79, 149
  design strategies to enhance, 76–8
  in corridors, 68–70, 85, 147
  in knowledge work, 58, 66–68
  in relation to designed space, 27, 34, 70–3, 81, 85–6
  with patients, 45,
    see also Spaces for Communication Index, (SCI)
community, 39, 46, 56–60, 80, 141–2
concurrent visibility, xxiv, 33–6, 38–40, 149
configuration, 37, 42, 64, 69–71, 134
copresence, 3, 6, 141
corridor, 15, 92–5, 142, 147
  and patient surveillance, 23, 29, 33, 39
  and nurse travel efficiency, 65–6
  appearance of, 108–9, 111–113, 115–16, 149
  communication and collaboration in, 55, 68–9, 73, 76–9, 82, 85
  guidelines for design of, 99, 105–6, 144
  in COVID-19 hospitals, 134, 139, 143
  navigation and wayfinding in, 97, 100, 104–7
  signage and graphics for, 120, 124
COVID-19, 45, 73, 130–143, 146, 148

decentralised nursing, xxiii–xxiv, 39, 69, 76–78, 80–1
district, 107, 120, 122
division of labour, 58–60, 67
doctors, 56, 58–60, 66–70, 78–9, 147–8
Durkheim, Émile, 60

efficiency, 58, 60–67, 70, 80, 82–5, 110–112
empathy, 92, 109, 118–19, 143
encounter, 18, 32, 68–9, 79, 141,
evidence-based design, xxiii–xxv, 4–5, 23, 144–5, 148

family, 10, 25, 58, 73, 146–8
  presence of in hospitals, 41–7, 73, 94, 142
Fangcang shelter hospital, 135–6
field of view, 33–4,
  see also isovist
front stage, 67–8

gestalt, 99, 103–4
Goffman, Erving, 6, 67, 79, 95
graphics, 61, 92, 99, 104, 120–3

hallway, 1, 14–5, 78, 92–6, 105,
  See also corridor
Hanson, Julienne, xxii–xxiv, 147
Hillier, Bill, xxii–xxiv, 31, 141–2, 147–9
hippocampal map, 101–2
human-centred design process, 117–124
Huoshenshan emergency hospital, 133–5, 140

infection, xxiii, 73, 131, 133–6, 138, 140–3,
  see also sepsis
institution, 15, 32, 61, 92–5, 108–16, 120
integration, 5, 39, 81, 84, 98, 106,
  see also space syntax
intelligibility, xxv, 145
intensive care, 21, 37, 66, 131, 139–40, 146,
  see also acute care
interface, 147
isovist, 30–32, 34–41,
  see also field of view
isovist connectivity, 21, 34–42,
  see also space syntax

knowledge workers, 55, 58, 66–8, 70, 79

lobby, 96, 103, 109, 120

M. D. Anderson cancer center, 81
mental models, 102
monitoring, 25–6, 28–9, 34, 131,
  see also observation, patient,
  see also surveillance
mortality, 21–3, 28–33, 36–8, 61–2, 69, 133
movement, 30–6, 64, 68–71, 78, 85, 147
museum, 5, 32, 114

navigation, 95, 101, 104, 105–7, 132, 145

National Health Service Nightingale hospital, 138–40
Nightingale, Florence, 58, 60–2, 78
Northern Beaches Hospital, 120-7
Nuffield Provincial Hospitals Trust Studies, 4–7, 64
nurse practice, 26–7
nurse station, 23, 28–30, 33–4, 37, 39, 76, *see also* team station
nurse work, 4, 28, 44, 66–7, 70, 78
  history of, 60–2

observation, patient, 30, 43, 50, 69, *see also* surveillance, *see also* monitoring

pandemic, 41–5, 130–2, 137, 140–1, 143,150
patient head of bed, 32–3, 35–6, 38
patient room, 42–5, 65, 69, 112–3, 134
  layout properties on ward, 23, 27, 33, 38–39, 74
  nurse station location relative to, 44, 65, 81, 84
  single patient room, xxiii, 73–4, 140, 147
Peckham Experiment, 8, 10
Pioneer Health Centre, 8–10, 13
Privacy, 13, 39–42, 44–5, 73, 96
profession, 4, 58–61
Promedica medical center, 81-2
public health, xxiv, 117, 132, 148

route knowledge, 97–98

sepsis, 36, 38–40
solidarities, 60, 111, 136, 140–3
space syntax, x, 3, 5–6, 69, 105–6, 141–3, *see also* isovist connectivity, *see also* integration, *see also* visibility graph, *see also* visual connectivity
Spaces for Communication Index (SCI), 55, 70–8
Stanford hospital, 41–7
Surveillance, 8, 73, 94, 136, 149,
  in acute care, 23–30, 32–5, 39–40, 41–7, 60
Surgicenter, 10–13
survey knowledge, 97–8, 100

Taylor, Frederick, 63, 66
team performance, 26, 34, *see also* teamwork
team station, 25, 29, 33, 39, 81, *see also* nurse station
teamwork, 55, 58, 60, 67–8, *see also* team performance
ties, social, 141–3
transpatial, 141–2
travel distances, 44, 55, 65, 115
type,
  architectural, 3, 6–8, 13–14
  of inpatient unit, 37, 43, 62, 71, 74–5
  of hospital, 106, 108, 112, 135, 140, 147
  of user persona, 118–19

unit, 27, 37–38, 41–43, 65, 71–3, 80–86
  inpatient unit, 80–1, 147
user–centred design, 117–20, 124

viewsheds, 69, 72–9, 145
visibility, 27–8, 39, 41–5, 62, 69–71,
  accumulated, 55, 71–2, 85
  targeted, 32–4, 146
  see also concurrent visibility
visibility graph, 31–2, *see also* space syntax
visitor, 92, 94–7, 116
visual connectivity, 31, 34, 37, 74–8, *see also* space syntax

ward, 60–79, 112, 133–4, 139,
  inpatient ward, 15, 55, 65, 73, 94, 112
  see also unit
wayfinding, 92, 95, 103, 117–24
  guidelines for hospital corridor layout and design, 105–6
Wuhan COVID–19 hospitals, 133–6, 139, *see also* Huoshenshan emergency hospital, *see also* Fangcang shelter hospital

Yale Traffic Index, 4, 64–5, 70–2

www.ingramcontent.com/pod-product-compliance
Lightning Source LLC
LaVergne TN
LVHW052018300826
846742LV00020B/85